# JUST BEFORE YOU RETIRE

Simeon Terhemen Kaase

**Simeon Terhemen Kaase**

08036270443
terhemen19@gmail.com

Cover design by: Kaase

# CONTENTS


Title Page

Copyright

Dedication

ACKNOWLEDGEMENT

CHAPTER 1 — 5

CHAPTER 2 — 19

CHAPTER 3 — 43

CHAPTER 4 — 54

CHAPTER 5 — 65

CHAPTER 6 — 74

CHAPTER 7 — 82

CHAPTER 8 — 89

WORKS CITED — 101

About The Author — 105

ABOUT THE BOOK — 107

# ACKNOWLEDGEMENT

Though I desired to put down my thoughts into writing many years back, the inspiration became stronger during my contact with Solomon Okpa aka Ogapatapata of the WRITE-FOR-ME in 2021. Ogapatapata has mentored me so dear and I really appreciate him. My boss in the office, the Executive Director of the Fellowship of Christian Nurses, Nigeria (FCN), Peter Maji introduced me to the Write-For-Me Academy where Ogapatapata subjected me to write. I am highly indebted to Peter Maji. He always kept encouraging me when I was almost withdrawing from the rigorously uncompromised training. I am indebted to my basic class coach Anthony Ojie, Director of Training, Fellowship of Christian Nurses, Nigeria (FCN). I appreciate you for the basic knowledge.

My family stood with me all the period. During the Christmas and New Year breaks of 2022/2023, I devoted my time to make finishing touches to this book and they understood with me. I really appreciate.

I give thanks to all the retirees that volunteered information during interview. They are:

i.   Gimbiya Hannatu Dikko Awon
ii.  Da & Ngo Joel Dawang
iii. Rev. Hosea G. Buba
iv.  Elder & Mrs. Danjuma Dassah
v.   Rev. SP. Dastu, R. Ring-le (Still in active service)
vi.  DSP. Abraham Tativ

vii. Rev. Ishaya Manomi

viii.     Dr. Wesley Damar

ix.  Mr. Emmanuel Onwe Akpo

x.   Mr. Clifford M. Dalong

xi.  Hajiya Hadiza Dije Mafiyai

All of them have retired except Rev. SP. Dastu, R. Ring-le who had few years to retire as at the time of interview. They are all doing well and have established the fact that it is possible to live at your best even after retirement. May God be glorified through all of you you.

I really appreciate this team of colleagues for standing with me: Rev. Elisha D. Pam (Chairman, RCC Gyel), Rev. Solomon A. Challom, Rev. Mafeng Y. Pwol, Pst. Philip Nangil and Terhemba Ikpom to mention but a few for every support they rendered to me.

# JUST

# BEFORE YOU RETIRE

*By Simeon Terhemen Kaase*

*"You cannot build the future for the youth, but you can build the youth for the future."*

...Roosevelt

◆ ◆ ◆

# CHAPTER 1



## *INTRODUCTION*

Several reasons informed my voluntary retirement from the Nigeria Police Force in 2005 after seventeen years of meritorious service. Foremost of these was that, while serving in the Police Force, I observed that after retirement, police officers often end up living miserably; this invariably results in them not living for too long before their eventual demise. The few fortunate enough to collect their exit (or retirement) benefits sometimes become incapacitated due to some chronic or terminal illness occasioned by organ failure. In contrast, some others carry on with lives of self-pity, helplessness, and hopelessness.

As a naive young man in my early twenties, the thought of this alone scared me stiff enough that I was determined not to remain in the Police Force till retirement. For me, it was a decision I made to retire voluntarily while still strong and healthy. Therefore, I began to plan so I would not exit unprepared.

It is interesting to mention that my uncle, who facilitated my recruitment into the Force, died within two years of his retirement. It might also interest you that my father served in the Nigerian Army and later converted his service to the Nigeria

Police Force, retiring after serving for 35 years. He did not live long before he developed cardiac failure and passed on in 2013. All these further compounded my fears, even though I had already voluntarily exited.

As an inexperienced young man, I thought these service personnel were corrupt, according to the general belief or opinion, and hence, were reaping the fruit of their labor. Indeed, as a serving officer, I struggled to be different rather than tread the path of corruption, and this made me quite uncomfortable, at least with the officers around me. I refused to be mentored in that manner. Most of them appeared to have lost their sense of integrity to corrupt tendencies. This vice could be another reason I decided to disengage from service midway. Timothy Nwan, in his book titled **"The Integrity of a Name,"** asserts that *"A man of integrity must live a blameless life, a life of faithfulness, moral purity, discipline, self-control, live wisely, and have a good reputation."* I struggled to live a life of integrity to avoid being infected or, better yet, developing what I call the **"Human Integrity Deficiency Syndrome"** (HIDS).

Society perceived (in fact, still perceives) members of the Police Force to be so corrupt that nothing or no one could correct the notion. I could not even defend the same, being an eyewitness myself. I didn't know what was obtainable in other sectors of the economy; therefore, I concluded that I should stand with society.

I was born into a family of six, three boys and three girls. My late father, Inspector James Kaase Tyem (rtd.), was a devout Christian. My mother and grandmother were also devout Christians. Our parents instilled Christian values in the six of us; hence, we were morally sound and upright. I grew up to know Christ personally, and this background helped me to eschew evil. I detest and abstain from anything and everything evil. Therefore, I struggled to balance my Christian life with what I saw in the Nigeria Police Force. For me, it was indeed a real struggle. With this brief background, one can understand and see a young man struggling to live a righteous life without a mentor.

The Church, I mean the body of Christ, did not help matters. The moment they realize you are a member of the Police; they withdraw from you and keep their distance as much as possible. This is simply because of their preconceived notion that you are a corrupt fellow, a sinner.

Before I proceed, let me quickly state here that my thoughts on why Police officers retire and become incapacitated were utterly wrong. As I advanced in age and knowledge, I soon observed that civil servants generally only live for a short time after retirement. Could that also be a result of corruption? I will address this question and many others in this discourse.

The challenge isn't just peculiar to serving officers in the Police or military; therefore, my judgment about the Police was wrong. I later discovered that corruption and wickedness in the civil service surpass what we see in the police force. Regrettably, this includes even religious institutions.

Our concern here is not about corruption. Hence, let me bring my thought to a conclusion. The Police, in fact, the civil service in its entirety, and every other extraction of the society, be it social, economic, etc., is corrupt simply because the culture is corrupt, and the government of the day fans the flame of corruption. This is my opinion.

This book will examine why people retire and fail to live long again. They either develop one sickness they never recover from or remain perpetually poor. Some retirees do not even benefit from their children upon whom they have labored so much. Shall we say it is the plan or intention of God that people suffer in such a manner, even at retirement? We will look at the missing link and suggest a way forward toward enjoyment after service in old age, which I believe is God's intention for His children.

In the western world, people look forward to a happy retirement. The reverse is the case in Nigeria and third-world countries, where people are scared stiff each time the thought of retirement comes to their mind. They change their age repeatedly to enable them to remain in active service. However, there will be no hiding place when nature calls or when age tells on your body. As the famous saying goes, that one cannot cheat nature, Rev. Joshua Dayok describes retirement from active service as scriptural, citing Moses, Samuel, and many others as men of God who had to retire to give way for the younger ones to take over.

This book was meant originally for those in the Nursing profession as they prepare for retirement. Being a Nurse, I have been privileged to see how many retire and live hopelessly. As a Pastor, I thought this information would also come in handy for pastors alike as the same phenomena apply to them.

As God would have it, an ultimate direction came from above that this book should address everyone in all professions and aspects of human endeavor. This book speaks to civil servants, public servants, those in the Military, Police, and every security institution. The book also addresses traders, business people, farmers, students, etc. The reason for this is plausible; whatever it is you happen to engage in, someday, you must retire. The day comes when you cannot carry out those duties as you used to.

God Almighty is the only Being or Personality with no beginning nor end. For everything that you do, which has a start, indeed has an end, and no matter how long it takes, it will surely come someday. God Almighty, in His divine wisdom, planned and executed His work of creation logically and chose to rest on the seventh day. God used this to set an example to teach us that rest is crucial in life.

## Dsp Abraham Tativ

DSP Abraham Tativ has successfully disproved my opinion and

disabused my thought regarding this issue.

He is a retired Deputy Superintendent of Police resident in Gboko, Benue State (in the middle belt of Nigeria). He lives with his wife, Mrs. Esther Mbasughun Tativ, and four children. He was recruited into the Nigeria Police on September 1, 1975, and retired after 35 years of meritorious service on September 1, 2010. Throughout this period, he served in the Communications Department and retired as the Benue State Police Communications Officer. By implication, overtly or covertly, he was never involved in any form of corruption, as he had no access to the public.

## Plan For Retirement

DSP Abraham Tativ trained his wife at the College of Health Technology Mkar in Gboko.

He also went to the same College and graduated. It is worth mentioning that this Police Officer was recruited into the Police Force with Primary School Certificate. During his service, he studied and obtained his O' Level Certificate, which he used to secure admission into the College of Health Technology, Mkar, eight years before his retirement. He stated he was on night duty all through the years he spent in College studying. This is an articulate plan for retirement, though a challenging one. It was Bongos Ikwue and Ollie that said, "Nothing good comes easy."

## Retirement

At retirement, the couple now operates a standard private Hospital in Gboko. They also have a poultry farm. These two sources keep sustaining them during this period of retirement. The Association of Retired Police Officers Welfare, Gboko Chapter appointed DSP Abraham Tativ as their Treasurer because they know that their finances are safe, having known him with a clean record of faithfulness and accountability.

## Counsel

DSP Abraham Tativ counsels that everybody should know at the onset of starting any work that a day to retire is coming. They should plan to have their accommodation where they would retire and settle. They should marry in good time to train their children before they retire. They should also know that government will not care much for them in retirement. They should not rely on retirement benefits.

## Definition

Retirement can be defined as the beginning of new life, starting from the point of separation from active employment up to the point of death. It can also mean withdrawing from your position or occupation in which you have been through your active years.

By nature, every individual goes through a process of retirement in life. In Nigeria, the government's official retirement age is 60 years, which coincides with the natural retirement age. At this age, there is always physical, social, and mental retirement of activities. People tend to withdraw from most activities they naturally were used to while they were younger.

## Dr. Wesley Damar

Dr. Wesley Damar retired as a lecturer from the College of Agriculture Garkawa in Mikang Local Government, Plateau State,

Nigeria, in 2021. Before his retirement, he had set up his retirement plan and was running with it. He built his house where he lives with his family; his wife and three children. As an Agriculturalist, Dr. Damar has an orchard from which he supplies fruits to me personally. I met him on the farm, busy enjoying his work with his usual smile. He was relaxed. He is into crops and animal husbandry; he owns piggery, banana, and maize farms. He once told me fondly, "you don't pay transport going to work any longer. When you are working, there are expectations on you from people, friends, and relations. They would inundate you with demands because they know you are working, but when you retire, they know you are retired, and the demands will be less".

The major challenge with retirees is that the government needs to pay retirement benefits immediately. So, this does not go well with those who retire without anything to fall back on. If you regularly get your pension, you will live with minimal challenges. At the prime stage of your retirement, you can engage young people for labor and invest your benefits. At least five years after retirement, one should still be physically strong to supervise his work. When you are seventy and above, you may depend on other people to help you manage your work, according to Dr. Damar.

## Types Of Retirement

For this book, we will restrict the types of retirement to three.

- Traditional retirement
- Semi-retirement
- Temporary retirement

## Traditional Retirement

Traditionally, people retire from activities around 65 or so and stop working permanently. No part-time or full-time work anywhere. People at this point live on pensions or monthly Social

Security payments, which they have been able to earn by working all those decades.

It is this income, together with any retirement savings they accrued, they use to cater for bills and other expenses that may arise.

## Semi-Retirement

Semi-retirement is when, after a certain age, one continues to work in some capacity, usually part-time, rather than discontinuing work out rightly. This can mean anything from stepping down from your previous role at your place of employment and becoming a consultant or changing careers completely to do something you consider more meaningful or fun, aside from what you've been doing. This is my type of retirement from the Police Force years back.

With this type of retirement, you can supplement your retirement income while also remaining active at the same time. If you desire to keep moving daily or stay vibrant and relevant, semi-retirement is the answer.

Semi-retirement also allows you to transition to traditional full retirement once you feel you're physically, mentally and financially prepared.

## Temporary Retirement

Temporary retirement is characterized by working in a career for some time, retiring from that career for a brief period, and then returning to the workforce. It's a unique approach to retirement as it helps to prepare one for the reality that looms. It can be rewarding if you can afford to stay away from work.

It offers the flexibility to change careers or pick up where you left off, though this approach requires advanced financial planning.

(https://www.actsretirement.org/retirement-resources/ resources-advice/what-to-do-in-retirement/3-types-of- retirement/).

## Case Study Of Rev. Hosea G. Buba

In March 2022, the retired Rev. Hosea G. Buba and his wife, Hadiza, celebrated 50 years of togetherness and faithfulness in marriage. When I visited their country home in the Borno State Capital of Maiduguri, they still looked so young, strong, and healthy. He said he would still dedicate more time to serving God if he were to start life anew. He said they never had a child in their first six years of marriage. People severely bad-mouthed them and said all kinds of unthinkable things. Soon, God blessed them with a son they named Digwa Hosea Buba and four other children six years after Digwa's birth. This family is also blessed with seven grandchildren. Digwa became a Captain in the Nigerian Army but was declared missing in action during the Boko Haram confrontation in Gwoza, Borno State, Nigeria.

Rev. Hosea G. Buba's retirement is a typical example of traditional retirement. According to Victor Izekor, Rev. Hosea Buba served at the University of Maiduguri for 19 years as a Senior Health Superintendent, after which he retired. He finds more joy in serving in the Church. The Reverend gentleman reached the retirement age of 65 years and duly retired in 2017.

At retirement, Rev. Hosea has a Radio program on which he airs the word of God every Thursday on "Radio Dandal Kura," responding to listeners' calls and counselling converts. He routinely visits and supports the Internally Displaced Persons' (IDP) Camp in Borno State, making good use of every opportunity to serve the Lord and to impact humanity while also appreciating God for the life and health to help friends home and abroad. According to him, it has been a massive success without any regret.

I know Rev. Buba with that; he has a good personality and command of English, Hausa, and Kanuri. He speaks all these languages fluently. He is a man of peace and wouldn't be out of place if we refer to him as a man with no enemy.

## Case Study Of Hajiya Kadiza Mufuyai

Hajiya Hadiza Dije Mafiyai was born in Gindiri in 1961 to the family of Alhaji Haruna Kharatu and Hajiya Rukaiya Suleiman Kwankoso of Kano State. She got married in 1981 to the late Hon. G. M. Mafiyai, the Ubangari of Bokkos Local Government Area. The union was blessed with a son, Suleiman George Mafiyai, and a grandson Mafiyai Suleiman George (Angel).
Hajiya, as she is widely referred to, is a Professional Nurse who served with the Plateau State Hospitals Management Board and retired at General Hospital Mangu in 2013 at the Mandatory 35 years of Service to God and Humanity.

## Engagement At Retirement

Hajiya operates a Private Clinic (Hope Clinic) in Mangu. She is active in politics and was appointed Honorable Board Member twice by His Excellency Simon Bako Lalong, the Governor of Plateau State. "Nursing work is my divine call, passion, and heart's greatest desire. To care for the Total Man - Spirit, Soul, and Body is just my humble service to God and humanity," Hajiya asserts.
Hajiya became a Christian in August 1988 through the influence of a friend, Amina Abdullahi, now Mrs. Embu, and the Fellowship of Christian Nurses, Nigeria. "Even the perspective of my Nursing practice changed when I became a Christian Nurse," according to Hajiya.

Some people supported Hajiya and influenced her life so much. They include her late husband, Hon. G. M. Mafiyai, Mr. Suleiman G. Mafiyai, His Excellency Simon Bako Lalong, Hon Rachel Adanchin, Pst. Sunday Andong, Prof. Steven Mallo, Justice Longji, Hon. Sam Damla, Hon Ezekiel G. Laban, Bro. Chris Mature and James O. Gulesh, to mention a few.

Hajiya had the privilege of traveling to countries like Egypt, Ghana, the Benin Republic, Togo, Israel, Jordan, and the Philippines. However, she regrets that her father and Hajiya Nana Hamidu Bamaiyi, who trained her, are not alive to enjoy the fruits of their labor. Alhaji Zakaria Kashi Mangu, a pillar in her life, has also gone beyond.

## Ngo Victoria Yop Yaro Bot Davou

I got to know of Ngo Victoria Yaro only after her demise, but her testimony has gone far to encourage my life. She worked with Funnah Bakery, Bukuru, in Plateau State as a cashier and later as a staff member with Funnah Catering Services between 1968 and 1981. She served for 13 years, after which she established her Bakery/Catering Services in 1985. She owned Rayfield Bakery and earned the nickname *"Mama mai cake."* Ngo Victoria managed her catering services until 1998, when the Nigeria Police Force (Education Unit) employed her. She retired in 2010.

Anyone, whether educated or not, can learn a trade, and if determined, one can live a fulfilled life and raise people. Ngo Victoria 'raised' her children with her cake.

## Golden Principles Of Life

1. Always remember that you can grow without destroying others.
2. Always be conscious that you can pursue your dreams and aspirations without sabotaging others.

3. Always remember that nobody must go down for you to rise.

4. No one must be ashamed or disgraced to sustain your smile.

5. Know that while others are rising, you can also rise.

6. Remember that finding satisfaction in the pain of others will never bring you true happiness.

7. What you wish others is a prayer for yourself.

8. Become the good fire that genuinely lights up others, not one that ruins the joy, goodwill, and expectation of others.

9. Never take delight in causing pain or sponsoring the tears of another.

10. Allow the genuine FEAR OF GOD to guide your days, STRENGTHEN YOUR RELATIONSHIPS and SET YOUR COURSE.

These are the paths to true peace, lasting influence, and meaningful living!

*The Happiest People Don't Have the Best of Everything;
They Make the Best Of Everything.*

$$\blacklozenge \quad \blacklozenge \quad \blacklozenge$$

# CHAPTER 2



## Case Study Of Rev. Sp. Dastu, R. Ring-Le

Rev. SP. Dastu, R. Ring-le currently serves with the Nigeria Police Force as the Plateau State Intelligence Bureau (SIB) officer in charge. He is a psychologist, clergyman, and public servant.

## Plan For Retirement

Rev. Dastu has in place a sustainable retirement plan as follows:

1. **Investment in education** He has established schools that are doing well.
2. He has a rehabilitation center for rehabilitating and integrating drug addicts into society.
3. He's got several capacity-building programs.
4. He is into human development and psychological services.
5. He owns and operates the "Dastu Foundation Clinic" in

Jos.

When asked about his motivation, he said, "passion, interest, and intrinsic satisfaction." According to him, he wants to leave a legacy and desires to be a philanthropist.

EVEN IF I DON'T KNOW HOW TO DO IT, I ALWAYS KEEP TRYING<br>UNTIL I LEARN IT.

## Lessons

This Police Officer has already set the wheels in motion for his retirement. A few years from now, he will retire and find fulfillment in those things he has established. He will not be redundant; instead, he will actively manage his investments and continue his humanitarian work. People can key into their passion and start doing something that will help them even after retirement. It is also sufficient to mention that his wife, Mrs. Margaret R. Ring-le, and their five children are all engaged in this project and doing fine.

There is a well-known saying that everything with a beginning must also have an end. Rev. Datsu was asked, *"When should you start preparing for retirement?"* The response was very unequivocal. Preparation for retirement ought to begin the day you receive your appointment letter. As absurd as this may sound, that is the correct answer, or, should I say, the sensible thing to do, though this is rarely the case. Time flies: 35 years will soon pass away, just like 35 days, and people are caught unawares. So, all things being equal, the individual should start preparing as soon as he starts the job, assuming that the individual in question has the prerequisite knowledge about the significance of planning for retirement.

If the individual is self-employed, as soon as he realizes his earnings, either in business or in whichever career he chooses, he must set the retirement plans in motion. Richard Dare Ajiboye says, and I quote, *"Your plan today helps you to have a mental picture of what the future may hold, but a plan only becomes a reality when it rides on the wheels of vision, backed with action."*

While you plan, remember that you will need more money in retirement than usual. All it takes is consistent learning; regular savings (set up an automatic savings deduction). Automatic deductions create a commitment to your financial future that helps you remember to save regularly. If you are serious about retirement, this is a significant step to give you some money you may need to spend or invest.

Get a personal financial advisor who can help you at this stage, work with you for a few months, and focus on building a savings and investment portfolio for you at your own pace. Once you get it right, it will be a walkover for you.

As the saying goes, "Whenever one wakes up, that is your *morning*." Note that this is your journey, not anyone else's. There are things you should keep in mind. Don't compare yourself with anyone. Start planning now, and don't procrastinate.

Please give yourself a TARGET and make sure it is a SMART one. This acronym means that your target should be **Simple**, **Measurable**, **Achievable**, **Relevant**, and **Time-bound**. You tend to feel under pressure to make up for the lost time, especially when you think time is no longer on your side. Let me issue a warning here not to fall into that pressure trap.

## Good Versus Evil

The quest to pursue good should be the priority of any person who wants to retire active and healthy. For anyone who desires to end well, the pursuit of good is a necessary tool. It is appointed for one to live once on earth. The quality of life that one leads is the most important thing.

Good is pure, and it's eternal, while evil is not, and it's temporal.

Evil endamages the good to exist. Sin does not exist on its own. Good is natural, while evil is artificial. The source of good is God. The focus of evil is self-satisfaction, while the focus of good is satisfying others.

## 20 Potentials That Will Pay You At Retirement

1. Potential to stay optimistic.
2. Potential to sell and negotiate.
3. Potential to speak to a large audience.
4. Potential to convey what you think and feel.
5. Potential to keep trying after a series of failures.
6. Potential to break a complex process down to pieces.
7. Potential to do things irrespective of the situation.
8. Potential to save and invest money.
9. Potential to shut up, listen and learn from others.
10. Potential to read, understand and memorize.
11. Potential to self-analysis.
12. Potential to understand what others feel.
13. Potential to learn how to learn.
14. Potential to walk away.
15. Potential to adapt, improvise, and overcome obstacles.
16. Potential to manage time effectively.
17. Potential to master your thoughts.
18. Potential to make decisions based on facts rather than emotions.
19. Potential to ask for help when necessary.
20. Potential to write words to persuade and influence others.

## Signposts To Success

God has made a lot of investments in us. He intends that

we should take advantage of these investments and grow our economy to make a successful living. He wants all creatures to live a joyful life. When there is a deviation from God's original plan for human beings, they risk groaning and failure. God's plan is for you to work, and Alexander Usman says *that poverty is sometimes a result of laziness. The Bible forbids laziness. Poverty is a choice because if you refuse to work, you invite poverty. The Bible admonishes that lazy people should go and learn from the ants:* ***"Go to the ants, you sluggard (lazy bones) consider its ways and be wise*** *(Proverbs 6:6)"*. As you work hard, apply wisdom.

God has given us life. The saying goes, "When there is life, there is hope." As long as we are alive, we are supposed to work while we can; that is, while it is still day. Once the day is gone, night falls, and when the energy is not there again, there is no more strength to achieve or do much.

A rich man's farm brought forth so much, and he proposed to pull down his storehouse since it had become too small to accommodate the bumper harvest; hence, he decided to build bigger ones to store his harvest. That night, God demanded his life. Life is not meant to be stagnant.

One reason people retire and die early is that they never envisage anything to do again. God created you to impact lives; that is what He expects from you. When life becomes stagnant, it is no longer meaningful. No matter your age, there should be something you desire in life. Humans should not exist solely to eat and sleep but to focus on something. There is no point in deciding not to work again because you have enough. If you reach this point of not working again, it means you have begun to dig your grave. This is what many people fail to understand. Jeff Bezos, the CEO of Amazon, could decide not to work again because he is the wealthiest man in the world. Aliko Dangote, the richest man in Africa, hardly sleeps, yet he has all it takes to sleep 24/7. Have you wondered why even the rich never stop working? It is because there is always a target.

Time is another resource that God has graciously gifted to all humanity equally. We have 24 hours a day, and everybody has to work or achieve whatever they have to while on earth. Success depends on how you make use of this 'limited' time. Time is precious and, when lost, cannot be recovered. You can never recover the time you have lost to worry or anxiety, inappropriate relationships, laziness, giving excuses, and pursuing frivolities.

God has endowed us with diverse kinds of gifts. Your gift may be different from your friend's, making you unique. What your friend does or would do to become successful differs from what you would have to do. A young man met me and shared how he met a long-time classmate and friend. They had lost contact for many years, and the friend appeared to be doing well. The friend later told him that he was into 'school runs.' This young man also wanted to follow suit and do the same thing his old friend did. I had to caution him about his wrong motive. He was acting based on his emotions. It should come out of passion if you want to run a school or do any other business. You should count the cost, plan well, and do a proper consultation. Firstly, his discipline was neither education nor education related. Secondly, there must be a passion for running a business or a school. I knew his friend's good looks alone were his drive. He had no passion for running a school or managing other people's children. He didn't ask his friend to tell him of the challenges he had been through to get to that stage.

Identify your God-given gifts and talents. This talent is the ability to work on a task or project with passion and less stress. You will not struggle when you identify your gift; you will not struggle but do excellently well. Others will struggle and lament, while you will find pleasure in doing it because it is your gift.

Are you talented in any way? Are there things you love to do and achieve with ease? Nurture those talents, exploit them, and don't give up. even when you encounter setbacks and don't give up on your dreams, if you give up, when you become older, you will look at your peers who stuck to and followed their passion and have excelled, and you will think to yourself, "That could have been me." Pursue a career, study a course you love. Don't waste years of your life in a field in which you find no fulfillment.

The grace of God is another signpost to success and a resource. Grace is a disposition of kindness, compassion, and goodwill from God. When God says yes to you, no one will dispute it. Grace is a state of divine influence and favor from God. When you find favor in God's eyes, He makes you succeed in everything you do. If you want to succeed in life, locate the grace of God.

God's promise is another investment He has made in humanity, including you. Our God is not wicked. His plans for you are good. He is a dependable God. Depend on Him; His promises will come to pass concerning you. His faithfulness is for everyone who believes in Him.

Some opportunities are signposts for success. Opportunity is a source of investment from God. Opportunities abound everywhere, but often we don't see them. Someone said that POOR means *Passing Over Opportunities Repeatedly*. Some people remain poor because they have missed opportunities several times. At their most exuberant age, some people neglected or ignored many doors that opened for them. Sometimes it is due to fear, laziness, or even pride, yet that was the best time for them to start a venture that would prepare them for retirement.

I detest poverty the same way I dislike hell. Solomon Okpa, aka *Ogapatapata* of WRITE-FOR-ME, hates poverty, evil, wickedness, pride, laziness, procrastination, gossip, and the like. *Ogapatapata* fights against poverty, oppression, suppression – gaslighting (POSG).

During your productive years, are you privileged to stumble on wealth early in life? Don't lavish it away in clubs, wasteful shopping, or riotous living. Commit the funds to profitable investments, widen your revenue stream, make that money work for you and keep it to take care of you in your later years.

## The Need For Early Preparation

Retirement planning starts with thinking about your retirement goals and how long you must meet them. Never postpone your planning for retirement to a later date.

Start planning for retirement as soon as possible to take advantage of the power of compounding interest. Younger investors can take more risks with their investments, while investors closer to retirement should be more conservative.

Retirement does not always turn out how people think it should because many believe that the future is automatically secured. Meanwhile, some are still figuring out what to do to retire comfortably. Sometimes it takes a long time for others to align with their new state of life, which the death of a spouse may alter, mortgage payment, change in eating habits, change in living conditions, education for grandchildren, and a whole lot more.

Generally, the older you get, the more your portfolio should focus on income and preserving your money. At this stage, you should invest in less risky investments, which may give you less proceed or dividends but will be less volatile and provide income that you can use to live on and less concerned about inflation. A 60-year-old planning on retiring next year does not have the same issues about a rising cost of living as a much younger professional who has just started working.

You may also need more money to purchase a home or fund your children's education at retirement. You must factor this outlay into the overall retirement plan. Try updating your plan once a year to keep your savings on track

You can improve Retirement planning accuracy by specifying and estimating early retirement activities, accounting for unexpected expenses in middle retirement, and forecasting other costs like medical costs. Also, consider Health insurance during planning for retirement. This will take care of unforeseen ailments that may come up in old age. You don't need to add financial stress to health challenges.

Planning and preparation are of utmost importance in all aspects of human endeavors. It is crucial and desirous, especially if one does not want to end up with failure because "he who fails to plan has planned to fail." Planning is, therefore, necessary to escape possible mistakes in the implementation process of an endeavor. If you want a peaceful and healthy retirement, then planning and preparation are non-negotiable.

A Church worker, Mr. Niya Karasu, with the Church of Christ In Nations (COCIN), retired early in 2022 after 25 years of service in Maiduguri, Borno State, Nigeria (Victor, Izekor). During his retirement service, his Pastor, Rev. James Ibrahim, described it as unfortunate that the mere mention of retirement provokes fear and anxiety in many because of poor preparation and uncertainty. He reminded the congregation of the need for early preparation for retirement since it is a phase people must face as long as they live.

Rev. James asserts, *"let us not assume that retirement or old age means that you are already spent or useless in the community because it avails the retiree the opportunity to rest, advice, and contribute meaningfully towards the development of the society. This is the time to put in motion your initiatives and explore other areas you were not opportune to while you were an employee. Through this, you could become an employer or self-employed"*.

In a related development, Rev. Mudinka Seri reiterated that retirement allows one to reflect on life and allows the younger ones to take over.

Rev. Dr. Obed Dashen, who happened to be the Vice President of The Church Of Christ In Nations, and his wife, Mrs. Tarphena Dashen retired from active service in 2021 (Timothy Alamba).

At the retirement service, the guest preacher, Rev. Dr. David Pofi (rtd), said that not all that starts well and that finishing well is a function of people's deliberate choices. It is, therefore, a duty that people should be intentional in planning for retirement.

> *"As long as the earth endures, seedtime and harvest, cold and heat, summer*
> *and winter, day and night, will never cease."*

Genesis 8:22 (NIV)

The Church can sensitize Pastors to prepare for retirement as soon as they are employed. The Church can review the policy of waiting until they have five years to retire (as reported by Joel Gomiyar) before preparing them for a seminar. Early preparation can serve them better.

Look at this one-year saving plan below:

| | | |
|---|---|---|
| Week 1 $10 | Week 19 $190 | Week 37 $370 |
| Week 2 $20 | Week 20 $200 | Week 38 $380 |
| Week 3 $30 | Week 21 $210 | Week 39 $390 |
| Week 4 $40 | Week 22 $220 | Week 40 $400 |
| Week 5 $50 | Week 23 $230 | Week 41 $410 |
| Week 6 $60 | Week 24 $240 | Week 42 $420 |
| Week 7 $70 | Week 25 $250 | Week 43 $430 |
| Week 8 $80 | Week 26 $260 | Week 44 $440 |
| Week 9 $90 | Week 27 $270 | Week 45 $450 |
| Week 10 $100 | Week 28 $280 | Week 46 $460 |
| Week 11 $110 | Week 29 $290 | Week 47 $470 |
| Week 12 $120 | Week 30 $300 | Week 48 $480 |
| Week 13 $130 | Week 31 $310 | Week 49 $490 |
| Week 14 $140 | Week 32 $320 | Week 50 $500 |
| Week 15 $150 | Week 33 $330 | Week 51 $510 |
| Week 16 $160 | Week 34 $340 | Week 52 $520 |
| Week 17 $170 | Week 35 $350 | |
| Week 18 $180 | Week 36 $360 | |

$520 is enough to invest in a small business that can sustain you at retirement. The amount to save here depends on how things are for you and also your income.

## Reasons You Should Save Money.

### 1. The Habit of Saving

Everyone must embrace the habit of saving, particularly on rainy days. It is a discipline that can deliver you from shame at retirement or even before retirement. If you choose to start small, make it a sustainable habit. This saving should be in a separate account. Most individuals don't have the discipline to save. What they are very good at is spending. Some people want to save but lack self-discipline. Learning to keep a small amount of money will help cultivate financial discipline.

Isaac O. Ijaopo says savings are a reliable and formidable source of family funds to start a family business and to avoid borrowing. He admonishes that people should start saving in any possible way.

## 2. Investment

Rebecca Samuel Dali defines investment as "what you receive in return for contributing a resource. Furthermore, investment is expected to provide a future benefit that exceeds the value of the resources given in exchange". The most important reason you should save is wealth accumulation through investment. Make an investment budget where you put in money specifically for investment. Keep monitoring it continuously and as soon as it reaches the target for the business of your choice, then invest.

Different investments may be viable; however, you must involve experts to guide you correctly so that you invest wisely. Investment in mutual funds, shares, and bonds are other ways to diversify your funds and a profitable approach to verify your retirement plan. Investors should use wisdom in choosing where and how to invest.

You will need an expert to manage your retirement portfolio in a related development. This expert management is rare in Africa, but it pays. The person is experienced and can control your funding portfolio, using vital methods to develop your retirement financial savings.

You can equally check on many other techniques for investment yourself. There are newspapers, podcasts, and apps that expose you to available markets and choices.

Robert Kiyosaki shared three basic rules of investment in one of his books. These rules are simply talking about savings and investment.

a. Always know what kind of income your work generates.

b. Convert earned income into a portfolio or passive income as efficiently as possible.

c. Keep your earned income secure by purchasing security you hope to convert your earnings into passive income or portfolio income.

## 3. To Make A Huge Purchase

Assuming you want to make a capital purchase, say a plot of land worth $1,000, you earn just $200 every month.

There is no way you can afford it. You need to start a monthly savings of the amount convenient for you. Here is a simple calculation for 30% monthly savings:

30% of $200 = $60

60 x 18 months = $1,080

You can save it up in 18 months.

That means you plan to purchase the plot of land within two years.

Note: the percentage depends on how convenient things are for you and your income.

## 4. Unexpected Expenses

Plan to set aside emergency funds account. In Africa, many things will always come, particularly from extended family. You must take care of these needs.

## 5. Steer Clear Of Impulse Purchasing

Some time ago, my friend and I were driving down the city. He saw a DVD case and thought it was a Bible case. He hurriedly beckoned the hawker in the traffic and quickly made payment even when I advised against it. He did not plan to buy it then, but he got carried away. We got home, and he discovered he didn't need what he had bought. People sometimes get to regret their actions merely because they made impulsive purchases. To assist you, list what you want to buy before going out. Decide to avoid an impulsive purchase.

## 6. Dispose Of Properties Not Needed

Whatever you have in the house that is no more useful to you, please discard them. There are people around that can always buy them off as scraps. These worthless materials occupy space in the house and make your home unkempt. They become junk and useless. These could be unrepaired cars kept on blocks for years and could be electronics, furniture, or kitchen utensils.

## 7. Purchase In Bulk

Purchasing in bulk is cheaper. It saves you a lot of money. Non-perishable foodstuffs such as rice and beans are better bought in size since they can last long.

## 8. Take Public Transport

It is cheaper and healthier to take public transport sometimes. This can save what you will be spending on car maintenance and fueling. With wisdom and caution, you will channel the money into your savings account for tomorrow. In addition, it serves as a form of exercise for you. Experts have told us that aging begins from the feet up and an excellent way to keep fit in old age is by walking enough.

## Avoid Making Too Many Mistakes

There are mistakes people make in life that they later live to regret in old age. I will discuss some of the errors here for readers to learn. When younger, we make various choices without the future in mind. Sometimes those choices bite us in our mid-life. These are some of the things one might regret as one gets older.

Avoid procrastination. Whatever you are convinced to do in life, go ahead and do it. People may have opinions about you, particularly about your capability to deliver. However, once you are convinced, forget whatever the people say. Learn to believe in yourself, and don't doubt your ability to perform.

Don't exaggerate things. Sometimes there are challenges in life that may be overwhelming. However, it would be best to trust your ability to overcome. In reality, Goliath was bigger than David, but David trusted in God, and because of his previous experience, he faced the giant and defeated him. As you face a difficult situation, avoid anxiety, remain calm and resolute, and think appropriately about how to approach the matter.

<u>Don't allow others to rule and dictate your life or control you</u>. People can toss you here and there. They may expect you to do more than you are doing but run at your pace. Everyone has a divine assignment on earth. Allow them to pursue their assignments and concentrate on their own. Your destiny is different from theirs. For instance, somebody may say that in your community, there is no Lawyer; therefore, you should go and read law, whereas your strength is Physics. Please pursue your heart's desire.

<u>Don't rush into marriage because all your friends or mates are now married</u>. Also, don't marry someone for reasons other than companionship. Again, marry somebody that you are compatible and comfortable with; that is why there is time for courtship to enable you to study and get acquainted with each other. Don't misinterpret the famous saying, "look before you leap," as getting married late. Marrying late has its repercussion too. While you are still young, check your motives for getting married. Don't marry out of pressure or for social standing. Instead, marry for love and companionship, get married to the right person, and marry your best friend. If you get married to the wrong person or for the wrong reasons, you might live to regret it as you would have to put up with that person for the rest of your life. Things might get worse between you two; then depression, physical abuse, extramarital affairs, pain, shame, court cases, and bitterness, to mention a few, will define your mid-life years all because you chose the wrong person. Things would get worse when children are involved. Make the right choice of a spouse when you are young.

When people are younger, they care little about relationships. Most people think about getting money and moving up the ladder of success at all costs. Many use and trample on people to progress. They take relationships for granted, messing up bonds and sleeping around for personal gain. But these wrong actions will catch up with you ahead when you realize how empty life is without love and friends. You may have success at this time, but nobody to confide in. Worse still, you may be poor, and no one will be available to help you.

You are a young lady, and you became pregnant and got scared. You opt for abortion; years later, you will look back and wish you had kept that baby. More painfully, if fortune smiles on you, you will wish that child you gave up on is around to enjoy the fruits of your hard work. Being a single mother doesn't mean you can't make headway in life or that you wouldn't find a man in the future. Two young people decided to go for the option of abortion during their courtship. They later got married but were never able to have a child again until old age caught up with them.

Don't let your fears overcome you. Everybody has some degree of anxiety. However, when fear becomes excessive, it hinders success. Exercise faith when making significant decisions in life; else, you cannot progress. If you notice a good portfolio for investment, take the risk and invest. Investment is risk-taking. Someone rightly said that it is risky not to take a chance.

You become wiser when you are much older, and God becomes more real as you see life more meaningfully. But don't wait to get older to start enjoying a relationship with God. Know God when you are young and build your future with God. Don't be a young rebel who only returns to God when age catches up.

When you are older, a legacy is critical. The value of your name is crucial. You will ask yourself what your reputation is. What are you leaving behind? Your legacy is the total of your actions since your youthful days. We write our biography by how we live life every day. When you look back on your path and see the mud you threw at your name, the shame you attracted, and the little value you have added to the world, you will regret it.

You have only one body to live with all your life. The cigarettes, the alcohol you abuse, the drugs you take, the unhealthy foods you're fond of consuming; all that will destroy you slowly. When you are 50 and lifestyle diseases catch up with you, you will wish you had cared better for your body while you were much younger.

When younger, it is easy to show contempt to your parents; what do your parents know? They are old-fashioned, shady, and small-minded. But your parents are still your parents whether you agree with them or not, whatever their style. Don't wait for your parents to die or get separated from you before you think of reconciling or making up. When you get older, you will realize why your parents wanted to be close to you. The older you get, the more you see the value.

Is there that great person in your life loving you well? Don't repel or push that person away, or else they will walk out of your life, and you may never find them or their type. Don't wait to allow yourself to live in regrets of if only I had known, I would have held on to that person.

## Avoid Alcohol. See 75 Biblical Truths About Alcohol.

1. Genesis 9:20-26 - Noah became drunk; the result was immorality and family trouble.
2. Genesis 19:30-38 – Lot was so drunk he did not know what he was doing; this led to immorality.
3. Leviticus 10:9-11 – God commanded priests not to drink

so that they could tell the difference between the holy and the unholy.

4. Numbers 6:3 – The Nazarites were told to eat or drink nothing from the grapevine.

5. Deuteronomy 21:20 – A drunken son was stubborn and rebellious.

6. Deuteronomy 29:5-6 – God gave no grape juice to Israel, nor did they have intoxicating drink in the wilderness.

7. Deuteronomy 32:33 – Intoxicating wine is like the poison of serpents, the cruel venom of asps.

8. Judges 13:4, 7, 14 – Samson was to be a Nazarite for life. God sent the angel to tell his mother not to drink wine or a strong drink.

9. 1 Samuel 1:14-15 – Accused, Hannah said she drank no wine.

10. 1 Samuel 25:32-38 – Nabal died after a drinking spree.

11. 2 Samuel 11:13 – David hoped to cover his sin by getting Uriah drunk.

12. 2 Samuel 13:28-29 – Amnon was drunk when he was killed.

13. 1 Kings 16:8-10 – The king drank himself into drunkenness when assassinated.

14. 1 Kings 20:12-21 – Ben-Hadad and 32 other kings were drinking when they were attacked and defeated by the Israelites.

15. Esther 1:5-12 – The king gave each one all the drinks he wanted. The king was intoxicated when he commanded the queen to come.

16. Psalm 75:8 – The Lord's anger is pictured as mixed wine poured and drunk by the wicked.

17. Proverbs 4:17 – Alcoholic drink is called the wine of violence.

18. Proverbs 20:1 – Wine is a mocker, strong drink is raging.

19. Proverbs 23:19-20 – A wise person will not be among the drinkers of alcoholic beverages.

20. Proverbs 23:21 – Drunkenness causes poverty.

21. Proverbs 23:29-30 – Drinking causes woe, sorrow, fighting, babbling, wounds without cause, and red eyes.
22. Proverbs 23:31 – God instructs not to look at intoxicating drinks.
23. Proverbs 23:32 – Alcoholic drinks bite like a serpent, sting like an adder.
24. Proverbs 23:33 – Alcohol causes the drinker to have strange and adulterous thoughts, produces wilfulness, and prevents reformation.
25. Proverbs 23:34 – Alcohol makes the drinker unstable.
26. Proverbs 23:35 – Alcohol makes the drinker insensitive to pain, so he does not perceive it as a warning. Alcohol is habit forming.
27. Proverb 31:4-5 – Kings, princes, and others who rule and judge must not drink alcohol. Alcohol perverts good judgment.
28. Proverbs 31:6-7 – Strong drink could be given to those about to perish or those in pain. Better anaesthetics are available today.
29. Ecclesiastes 2:3 – The king tried everything, including the intoxicating drink, to see if it sufficed, yet it did not. (Ecclesiastes 12:8)
30. Ecclesiastes 10:17 – A land is blessed when its leaders do not drink.
31. Isaiah 5:11-12 – Woe to those who get up early to drink and stay up late at night to get drunk.
32. Isaiah 5:22 – Woe to "champion" drinkers and "experts" at mixing drinks.
33. Isaiah 19:14 – Drunken men stagger in their vomit.
34. Isaiah 22:12-13 – The Israelites choose to drink; their future looks hopeless.
35. Isaiah 24:9 – Drinkers cannot escape the consequences when God judges.
36. Isaiah 28:1 – God pronounces woe on the drunkards of Ephraim.
37. Isaiah 28:3 – Proud drunkards shall be trodden down.

38. Isaiah 28:7 – Priests and prophets stagger and reel from beer and wine, err in vision, and stumble in judgment.
39. Isaiah 28:8 – Drinkers' tables are covered with vomit and filth.
40. Isaiah 56:9-12 – Drinkers seek their gain and expect tomorrow to be like today.
41. Jeremiah 35:2-14 – The Rechabites drank no grape juice or intoxicating wine and were blessed.
42. Ezekiel 44:21 – Again, God instructed the priests not to drink wine.
43. Daniel 1:5-17 – Daniel refused the king's intoxicating wine and was blessed for it along with his abstaining friends.
44. Daniel 5:1 – Belshazzar, ruler of Babylon, led his people in drinking.
45. Daniel 5:2-3 – The king, along with his nobles, wives, and concubines, drank from the goblets removed from God's temple.
46. Daniel 5:4 – Drinking wine was combined with praising false gods.
47. Daniel 5:23 – God sent word to Belshazzar that punishment would be swift for the evil he had committed.
48. Hosea 4:11 – Intoxicating wine takes away intelligence.
49. Hosea 7:5 – God reproves princes for drinking.
50. Joel 1:5 – Drunkards awake to see God's judgment.
51. Joel 3:3 – The enemy is judged for selling girls for wine.
52. Amos 2:8 – Unrighteous acts of Israel included the drinking of wine received for the payment of fines.
53. Amos 2:12 – Israel is condemned for forcing Nazarites to drink wine.
54. Micah 2:11 – Israelites are eager to follow false teachers who prophesy plenty of intoxicating drinks.
55. Nahum 1:10 – God will destroy the drunkards of Nineveh.
56. Habakkuk 2:5 – A man is betrayed by wine.

57. Habakkuk 2:15 – Woe to him that gives his neighbor a drink.
58. Habakkuk 2:16 – Drinking leads to shame.
59. Matthew 24:48-51 – A drinking servant is unprepared for his Lord's return.
60. Luke 1:15 – John the Baptist drank neither grape juice nor wine.
61. Luke 12:45 – Christ warned against drunkenness.
62. Luke 21:34 – Drunkenness will cause a person not to be ready for the Lord's return.
63. Romans 13:13 – Do not walk in drunkenness or immorality.
64. Romans 14:21 – Do not do anything that will hurt your testimony as a believer.
65. 1 Corinthians 5:11 – If a Christian brother is a drinker, do not associate with him.
66. 1 Corinthians 6:10 – Drunkards will not inherit the kingdom of God.
67. Galatians 5:21 – Acts of the sinful nature, such as drunkenness, will prohibit a person from inheriting the kingdom of God.
68. Ephesians 5:18 – In contrast to being drunk with wine, the believer must be filled with the spirit.
69. 1 Thessalonians 5:6-7 – Christians must be alert and self-controlled, belonging to the day. Drunkards belong to the night and darkness.
70. 1 Timothy 3:2-3 – Bishops (elders) are to be temperate, sober, and not near any wine.
71. 1 Timothy 3:8 – Deacons are to be worthy of respect and not drinkers.
72. 1 Timothy 3:11 – Deacons' wives are to be temperate and sober.
73. Titus 1:7-8 – An overseer is to be disciplined.
74. Titus 2:2-3 – The older men and women of the Church are to be temperate and not addicted to wine.
75. 1 Peter 4:3-4 – The past life of drunkenness and

carousing has no place in the Christian's life.

When you know that alcohol can embarrass you, why do you indulge in drinking? Is it a necessity for life?

**No drunkard shall inherit the Kingdom of God (1 COR 6.10)**

## Case Study Of Clifford M. Dalong

Clifford M. Dalong is a Nurse Anaesthetist. He retired on August 26, 2022, from the National Orthopaedic Hospital, Dala, in Kano State, Nigeria. He retired after attaining the statutory retirement age of 60 years. When asked what he is doing now, he said, "managing my patent medicine store." He got motivated to do this business in 2016 as part of his retirement preparation. *"I am passionate about it. The story behind my passion for patent medicine store operation started in 1988 when I was assisting a senior colleague in his medicine store."* Clifford said his major supporter is his wife. He married Mrs. Jane Jummai Dalong, and God blessed them with three children.

### Preparation for Retirement

Clifford Dalong said he had conceived about retirement right from the beginning of employment. He appreciates God for the success so far. *"My joy is when my clients give me good feedback about their treatment. I sometimes use the opportunity to share the gospel with them. I have no regrets."* he concluded.

*"There's no place like home if someone is looking ahead in order to avoid destructive surprise."*

-McDonald

# CHAPTER 3

*Phases of Retirement*

Retirement is a gradual withdrawal from active service, often unpleasant and unexpected. It is a transition that is not easy to accept in some parts of the world, including Nigeria, but it is factual and compulsory. Retirement can attract various emotions and concerns. This chapter navigates the stages of retirement and will help people understand the reality and plan for it.

The statutory retirement age in the federal civil service is 60 years or 35 years of service, depending on which one comes first.

There are necessary adjustments that you will need to observe so they can help you live longer, be stronger, and live meaningfully after retirement. When you understand and plan well, you will enjoy a healthy life at retirement and remain relevant, fruitful, and fulfilled.

I will discuss the stages to ensure a smooth transition.

## Phase 1: Pre-Retirement

This stage begins 5–15 years or more before the final disengagement. It is characterized by imagining a new life while planning. You wake up and no longer go to the usual place you used to render service. You no longer interact with colleagues at the regular workplace. At the month's end, you no longer hear that beautiful alert you used to hear or receive.

Apart from the physical structure you plan to have, which is good, you must also prepare emotionally. Making sure you have fun and find purpose in this stage of your life. During this transition period, you need to consider what will make you happy and fulfilled, one of which is to learn how to control your emotions.

This stage can be a time of excitement, anticipation, worry, and doubt, especially in the year or two before retirement. Anxiety sets in when people worry they won't save enough money for retirement.

## Phase 2: Retirement Events

This stage, also known as the liberation phase, includes excitement, relief, and freedom from the stress and responsibilities of everyday working life. This can last for more than one or two years. It is characterized by reconnecting with family, friends, and spouses, spending time on hobbies, traveling, and starting new businesses.

## Phase 3: Disenchantment

A feeling of disappointment characterizes this phase of retirement. There are adverse reactions to losing space and time, especially for a person who is always busy. People may end up feeling like something is missing in their lives. There is unusual excitement and hopelessness, and loneliness is another experience. If you don't address these appropriately, it may lead to depression.

## Phase 4: Reorientation

Reorientation is an incredibly challenging readjustment period that involves creating a new identity. It can take some time and effort to accomplish. But once you have built a new identity, you can gain a sense of closure from your working days and move on to enjoy retirement as it's meant to be enjoyed.

To avoid depression, you must find something that gives you a meaningful purpose later in life, such as pursuing a passion, volunteering, and adding new fun activities to your daily routine.

## Phase 5: Stability

This stage may start up to 15 years after the official start of retirement, and it's the final stage. Retirees in this stage are content and hopeful in their transition and will experience less depression and anxiety.

In this stage, retirees are settled into a fun and rewarding retirement lifestyle, doing things that make them feel fulfilled. They prioritize simplifying their lives and living relaxing lifestyles.

They may be prevalent health conditions during this stage. Hence, retirees focus on maintaining their health and independence, sometimes by moving to retirement communities where they can age in a place with access to healthcare, amenities, activities, and friends nearby.

While not every person will experience each stage as intensely or for the same amount of time as others, most retirees will experience this process in some form once they stop working.

Retirement comes with many emotions and worries, like

any significant life change. But you thoughtfully plan for your transition to take care of yourself both financially and emotionally. In that case, you can help ease the overwhelming emotions of this significant life transition and spend more time enjoying your new life to the fullest.

## Gimbiya, A Retired Teacher

Gimbiyan Matan Kachia, Mrs. Hannatu Dikko Awon is a traditional title holder. She retired from the civil service as a Deputy Director of the Federal Ministry of Education and Principal at Federal Government College Rubochi, Federal Capital City Abuja, in 2020. She served meritoriously for 35 years. Gimbiya is a resident of Kachia Local Government, Kaduna state, Nigeria. She is blessed with three children; the first two are already graduates.

Farming is the primary stake of Gimbiya for now. She produces ginger and does some petty trading. She does not appear like some other retirees that seek pity. She is instead a giver. Gimbiya is taking care of some extended family members who are now dependents. How does she cope? She said those who suffer after retirement and become helpless and hopeless are those who did not plan well for retirement. She said people should be focused and always know that one day, they will retire, and their salary will not be there again.

I was excited while sharing with Gimbiya. She appears like a minister of a country or an ambassador. The secret? She said, "Exercise." "Exercise at least four times a week." She also said people should maintain good relationships with others around them. Above all, people should be closer to their God, worshipping him in truth and spirit.

Health-wise, Gimbiya counsels that people should develop a good and healthy lifestyle and eating habits from a young age. They should be selective about what they eat and avoid eating junk. During my interaction with Gimbiya Hannatu, she repeatedly repeated that people should maintain good rest and exercise in old age. They should avoid alcohol and not abuse drugs. Other things to avoid, according to Gimbiya, include hypocrisy, gluttony, and selfishness. They should avoid these so they don't suffer the repercussions of old age.

Since her retirement, Gimbiya asserted that her pension has not been regular. Sometimes Governments delay pensions for about five months. It will be stressful if one retires and they are still paying children's school fees. With this, she says one should marry early in life so that the person will have their children early enough. The children will complete their primary education before retirement. At retirement, one should not pay school fees unless it is for other dependents, as in a communal African society.

Gimbiya counsels that, to avoid stress, people should try to own their homes before they retire. Some civil servants are privileged to secure government quarters and sometimes feel comfortable and relaxed. They don't plan to build their own homes. This is a stress risk. Even if you occupy government quarters, try to build your own where you plan to settle after retirement. Some civil servants rent accommodation all through 35 years of service; after retirement, they continue to pay rent. This risk will add to stress and other related health hazards like hypertension, diabetes, arthritis, and ulcers.

## Self-Respect

It is good to be mindful of the lifestyle and habits that earn your respect before other people, even in retirement, and we will discuss some of them here. These habits can promote healthy relationships and reputation. Remember that people respect you for what you do.

I. <u>Personal hygiene</u>: Personal hygiene is an essential aspect of our daily lives that can impact how others perceive us. Being deliberate about basic hygiene practices such as showering regularly, brushing your teeth, and wearing clean clothes can make people respect you.

II.   <u>Considerate behavior</u>: Being considerate of others is a fundamental aspect of social etiquette. Respect other people's boundaries. Be courteous; showing empathy can make people respect you.

III.   <u>Honesty</u>: Honesty is a critical virtue that most people highly respect. Lying, being untruthful, or being dishonest can damage trust and make people lose respect for you.

IV.   <u>Responsibility</u>: Taking responsibility for our actions and following through on commitments is essential for building trust and respect. Failure to meet deadlines, not fulfilling obligations, or being unreliable can make people lose respect for you.

V.   <u>Good Communication Skills</u>: Good communication skills are essential for building and maintaining relationships. Listening, hearing, and respecting other people's viewpoints while also trying to understand their worldviews will earn your respect. Inconsistency can make it difficult for others to trust and respect us. It's essential to be consistent in your words and actions and to follow through on your commitments.

VI.   <u>Respect other people's beliefs and values</u>: Respecting others' beliefs and values is essential to being a good human being. When you respect others' opinions or values, they will respect you.

VII.   <u>Personal growth</u>: Personal growth is essential to being a well-rounded individual. Seek new experiences or challenges. Never relent or stop learning new things.

VIII.   <u>Negative attitude</u>: A negative attitude can be contagious and affect those around you. A negative mindset can make it difficult for others to respect you and lead to strained relationships.

When you are mindful of these habits and try to change them, it can improve your relationships with people and increase the respect you receive from others. Remember that it's never too late to make positive changes in your life, and the effort you put into improving yourself can have a ripple effect on those around you.

## Happy Couple In Retirement

Da Joel Dawang lives in the cold city of Jos, Plateau State, Nigeria, with his wife, Ngo Sarah Joel Dawang, and their children. They have four biological children. I so much respect, cherish and admire this family. It's a family that fears God and respected in the neighborhood and around the Tin city of Jos. I have no regret meeting this couple at their retirement.

Da Joel Dawang retired from the civil service in 2014 after 35 years of active service. He served specifically on the Public Complaints Commission. The Elder still looks young, strong, and healthy almost ten years after retirement. He shared his secret with me:

- He knew from the onset that one day he would retire, so he started planning early enough. Therefore, early planning is essential.
- His state of mind was fashioned so that whatever he did, he always remembered that it would never remain the way it was. He made up his mind that he would retire happily. That was his goal.
- He began to work out to get his accommodation. He doesn't think using one's retirement benefits to build a house will be healthy. One should develop his house before retirement.
- He planned for the size of the family he could comfortably manage. One astonishing thing he mentioned is that he

never had more than one child in secondary school. One graduates from a tertiary institution before the other goes to secondary school. It was so because of the spacing they did while bearing children. This reduced the stress of paying cumulative school fees and allowed them to build houses.

- He also started thinking of a business he could manage at retirement to avoid stress. Elder Dawang believes that in retirement, you only need a company that will keep you moving around and not a stressful business that will wear you out.

**Health and Social Life:** Da, Joel Dawang, and his family registered with the National Health Insurance Authority (NHIA) and are enjoying the insurance services. He believes that everybody should register for health insurance to avoid embarrassment, especially when they need medical attention and there one cannot afford the medical bill. What about diet? Da Joel Dawang passionately said that people should be intentional with what they eat. He is selective in what he eats, and his wife is conscious of this.

For the avoidance of doubt, Da Joel Dawang is a reserved person. However, he believes in the power of interaction. Meet him from a good perspective, and you will not think he is reserved. One thing standing out very clearly about him is that he discusses issues, development, social life, and religion. He asserts, "I don't care about people's opinions concerning my actions. You park your car and trek, people will talk (laughter). So let them say anything they feel like. If you worry about what people say, you won't progress." Da Joel Dawang has his grinding engine and operates the grinding machine himself. He said when people come with anything to grind, he does it for them; if they don't come, it doesn't disturb his peace. He also has laundry services, but the children took over their business. Retirement should not come with a stigma. It is a phase of life that everybody should look forward to seeing.

**Marital Life:** Da Joel Dawang is blessed with a lively, lovely, and industrious wife, Ngo Sarah Joel Dawang, who also retired recently on January 1, 2022. There is no dull moment with her. She served in the Veterinary Service, Plateau State Government, and retired as Chief Animal Health Husbandry Technologist (CAHHT) at grade level 14. Ngo Sarah Joel Dawang, in her usual smile, asserts, "I was looking forward to my retirement, hoping for a private practice on my farm." She is into poultry farming and mixed farming, crops, and livestock. According to her, this business keeps her busy as she provides services to people. It also helps her remember her profession. At the time of this interaction, her retirement benefits were still unpaid, yet she was not stressed. She was still meeting the needs of the neighbor and other dependents.

This retired couple has one thing in common; always smiling and laughing, and charity is their uniting factor. It may interest you that this couple has other children they support besides their biological children. Their children are well-behaved and obedient. This is evident that this couple is affecting life.

*Success has so many friends, but failure is an orphan.*

◆ ◆ ◆

# CHAPTER 4

## *Common Diseases Among Older People*

There are changes in the body of a man or woman when he or she grows older; we will examine some of the changes and possible accompanying diseases.

Life is in season, and each season has pros and cons. At an older age, certain diseases are more prevalent. However, there are general tips to maintain, reverse, or prevent some of these diseases if you have them. Some of the common illnesses among the elderly also affect the younger generation.

. Diabetes is a problem and disease that primarily affects the elderly. You may know somebody dealing with this problem, or you may be the one. There is a way out.

Another problem that afflicts the elderly is arthritis. Arthritis is a kind of disease that affects the joints of the body. The shoulders, fingers, ankles, toes, and back were mostly affected. They are unable to walk properly because of arthritis. There are ways to prevent arthritis.

Insomnia is another disease that is common among the elderly.

It is the inability to sleep for an extended period. You wake up, and you sleep it off again. Several other diseases, including hypertension, can arise if one cannot sleep well for a long time.

Osteoporosis, which causes bone density loss, typically causes older people to bend. They're unable to walk straight anymore because of weak bones. They fall easily and fracture their bones because the bones are fragile.

Menopause is another problem common among the elderly, especially women. When a woman has crossed her childbearing age and no longer menstruates, many hormonal changes occur in her body, so she begins to experience many symptoms that she does not understand. It is more severe among women than among men. For women, it is called menopause. For men, it is called andropause.

As a person ages, their sexuality changes, and their general performance is reduced. For men, impotence kicks in as you age. Although men don't often feel the impact until a much later age, it is still a factor that needs to be considered. Additionally, you may find it more challenging to attain an erection; even when you do, it might not be as firm as it used to be in your younger years.

The bladder and urinary tract may also be affected. This is because the bladder often becomes less elastic as you grow older, raising a person's risk of urinary incontinence and difficulty holding urine. In men, issues such as prostate enlargement and cancer may set in, making it much harder for them to empty the bladder.

As people grow older, another problem they notice is a slow metabolism. Your ability to digest food and assimilate nutrients becomes weaker than when you were younger. You will not discover that you can no longer accommodate three meals per day. You just became heavy because the food didn't digest quickly. When you understand that the rate of digestion slows with age, you will begin to reduce the number of times you eat to once or twice a day. That will be enough to sustain you instead of eating breakfast, lunch, and dinner.

George H. Malkmus believes that people should refrain from caffeine at an older age. According to him, "coffee is not a food, but a poisonous, addictive drug that can only do great harm to the body while being incapable of doing it any good."

There is an alteration in the digestive system in old age due to structural changes in the large intestine that result in higher chances of having constipation and many other digestion issues. Less activity, a lack of exercise, and a low-fiber diet threaten digestive problems.

Hypertension is usually terminal. It is more common among older people. However, living a life free of hypertension is possible, especially if you know the causes. My father died in 2013, and shortly after, I became hypertensive, as announced by the doctor. He prescribed a particular drug for me, but I refused to use the drug. Instead, I intensified my exercise, reduced my salt intake more reasonably, avoided eating late at night, and increased my intake of fruits and vegetables. What we need is not more medication but more education.

It's simply a change in the season of life accompanied by unpleasant symptoms that you can control if understood correctly. Therefore, as you age, there is a need for a change of lifestyle.

People 50 years of age and older are advised to change their lifestyles to avoid heart-related issues. At this age, the nerves stiffen and increase the risk of suffering from heat-related diseases like stroke.

Healthline recommends four lifestyles you should adopt when you are 50 years and above. During this period of your age, the organs in most people begin to weaken, and at the same time, their skin begins to wrinkle and look tired.

### 1. Don't Stress Yourself

The elderly should take the issue of stress very seriously. There is a relationship between stress and a wide array of health problems. Several studies have found that stress is associated with an increased risk of heart disease and altered blood pressure readings.

### 2. Stop staying up late at night.

The elderly should sleep between 7 and 9 hours per night. They place a high value on the time spent sleeping and relaxing. According to studies, older individuals should try to reduce their stress levels. This is because it is, from a medical point of view to their best advantage to do so.

### 3. Focus on eating more nutritious meals.

The elderly should restrict themselves from consuming potentially dangerous foods such as fast food and processed snacks. Instead, they should focus on consuming a diet that is more nutritionally sound and rich in fresh fruits, fiber, and vegetables.

### 4. Refrain from living a sedentary lifestyle.

Most older people, particularly those in poor health, would benefit from increased daily movement. This is because research has shown that leaving a sedentary lifestyle can have significant negative consequences on the overall health of the body.

It is dangerous to have a sedentary lifestyle since it increases the risk of developing heart disease, brain disorders, dementia, and stroke.

# Moringa Oleifera And Its Health Benefits

Moringa Oleifera is a plant with tiny leaves that promotes health and prevents disease, suffering, and death. Some sources say it is a native of India, while others say it was there in ancient times during the Greco-Roman world.

In the Hausa language, it is called Zogele Gandi. In the Igbo language, it is called Okwe-Oyibo. The Yoruba people call it Ewe-Ile or Ewe-Igbale. The Tiv people call it Jeghlegede, Igede-speaking people call it Iwowo, and Igalas call it Gerigedi.

When eaten fresh, the plant, also called "miracle tree" or "mother's friend," contains seven times the vitamin C of an orange. When the leaves are new, they have four times the vitamin A of carrots, while the dried leaves contain ten times as much of the vitamin.

The same leaves contain four times the calcium in milk when fresh, but when dry, they have 17 times as much calcium as milk. The potassium content in fresh Moringa leaves is three times the quality of the mineral in a banana, compared to 15 times when the leaves are dry. The leaves contain three times the iron in spinach, but the iron content is 25 times higher when dry. As for protein, the content is two times what you get in yogurt, but when it's dry, it is nine times more (Lowell Fuglie, 2001).

Ancient medicine has it that moringa can prevent about 300 diseases, while modern research has discovered about 539 nutrients in the plant (Moringarevealed.com).

Even in drier climates, this versatile plant can provide a stable, reliable food source; additionally, the high protein and nutritional content offer superior dietary value in areas where other forms of protein and amino acids are difficult to obtain. In remote communities where medical supplies and support are at a premium, the pharmaceutical quality of the seed, pods, and leaves can be invaluable in treating and providing rapid responses to developing health problems. At the same time, even technologically advanced societies can benefit from the antioxidant and anticancer properties of the enzymes in the leaves and stems. Because the leaves retain much of their nutritional value even after being dried and stored for a prolonged period, you can preserve them for significant periods without modern refrigeration methods. These qualities make the Moringa tree one of the most critical tools in international efforts to promote the health and well-being of less developed nations and small rural communities in India, Africa, South America, and the world.

According to Moringaoleifera.com, "Moringa is a healer, food magician, beautician, and a plant with surprising water purification capabilities, a best friend and humanitarian who works for a little. It is one of the most valuable trees on earth.

Moringa contributes significantly to human and animal health; in many cases, it can mean the difference between life and death.

No adverse effects of daily consumption of Moringa leaves have ever been reported".

Further scientific research reveals that these tiny leaves, also called the "tree of life," have the potential for prevention and curing.

All parts of the Moringa Oleifera tree are edible, and humans have long consumed them (Fuglie 2001). Many uses of moringa include Human health, Life stock Fodder, Plant growth enhancer, Biogas, etc.

## Medicinal Benefits Of Moringa

It has been discovered that the health benefits of moringa are too numerous to mention. Moringa has been used for centuries by the Indians and many parts of Africa without side effects recorded. The World Health Organization (WHO) has also conducted scientific research and concluded that Moringa Oleifera is highly nutritional and medicinal. Some research findings are stated below:

1. *Immune system*: It boosts the immune system against opportunistic infections. Thus, in Zambia, Uganda, Kenya, and Senegal, the dried leaves are extensively used by people living with HIV/AIDS.

2. *Stress*: It helps to combat stress by acting as a natural energy booster. It provides a long-lasting energy boost when used regularly. This energy boost is not based on sugar but is sustained. People frequently report much more endurance at work, home, and play.

3. *Diabetes*: A leaf extract can lower blood sugar levels effectively. It is the most effective remedy for the control and treatment of diabetes.

4. *Hypertension*: An extract from the leaf also stabilizes blood pressure and helps lower it by cleansing impurities in the arteries and working against the buildup of cholesterol.

5. Antibiotic: Moringa is used to treat infections. Its antibiotic property is identified as pterygosperimin.

6. *Skin Treatment*: Moringa has great healing benefits for the skin. It has been used to cure cuts, scrapes, sores, rashes, cracks, and other signs of aging.

7. *Anti-inflammatory*: Moringa is an anti-inflammatory for healing wounds and is very effective in treating trauma-initiated chronic swelling. It also controls ulcers.

8. *Body Detoxification*: It helps remove toxins by helping the kidneys and liver function effectively. It acts as a coagulant, attaching itself to harmful materials and bacteria to remove them from the body.

9. *Pregnancy and Breastfeeding*: Moringa is helpful to both pregnant women and breastfeeding mothers. It can do much to preserve the mother's health and pass on strength to the fetus and nursing child. It also increases the milk

production of nursing mothers and makes it richer in calcium.

## Why We Need Moringa

- Due to farmers' use of chemicals, fertilizers, and pesticides, trace elements in the soil have been used up and are no longer in the foods we eat daily.

- We store and preserve our foods with chemicals, thereby poisoning the food.

- About 75% of people deliberately or unknowingly consume the kinds of foods that cause harm to their bodies (junk, fatty, and beef foods).

- Only one-fourth of the world's population is truly healthy.

- Our cooking methods destroy a large portion of the nutrients in our foods.

- Environmental pollution, metal and industrial gases, dust, and smoke inhalation cause toxins and metabolic garbage to accumulate in our bodies.

- Excessive consumption of carbohydrates and unbalanced diets.

- Our lifestyle and genetic makeup also cause diseases like heart disease. Diabetics, cancer, arthritis, stroke, infertility, HIV/AIDS, obesity, prostrate problems, etc., creep into our bodies.

- Excessive consumption of sugary drinks and foods.

- Alcohol and smoking deplete the body of valuable nutrients and cause cirrhosis of the liver, lung problems, coughing, and cancer.

Moringa Oleifera contains the necessary nutrients to keep our bodies fit and healthy. It gives the body what any other food cannot because of the above reasons. It can nourish the body, prevent disease, and correct anomalies in the body system.

It is nature's most nutritious superfood for energy and muscle growth, best for children and breastfeeding mothers, and suitable for diabetic and hypertensive patients. It provides mental and emotional well-being, anti-aging, clarity, focus, and concentration, among others.

## Case Study Of Elder & Mrs. Danjuma Dassah

I met Elder Danjuma Dassah at his residence in Jos, enjoying his vegetable diet. Baba and Mama Rifkatu Dassah are enjoying good health ten years after retirement. Two were classmates at the College of Nursing, Vom, in Plateau State, Nigeria. They have been married for 42 years and have had four biological children. They could only remember some of the dependents they had raised and were raising. They had grandchildren living with them too.

The couple retired in 2012 after 35 years of service. Until their retirement, Elder Danjuma Dassah taught at the College of Nursing, Vom, while Mama Rifkatu Dassah served with the Pankshin Local Government Health Department. They both retired and did well, enjoying their retirement lives.

What are they doing? This couple, at retirement, is into mixed farming: crops and poultry farms. They started this preparation in 1986 while working closely but casually with Faith and Farm, a project of the Church of Christ in Nations (COCIN). Elder Danjuma learned how to keep chickens then, and the knowledge is helping them to this day. Every knowledge acquired in life while growing is not a waste.

Elder Danjuma said he used to take drugs to his village to carry out some treatment and help people. However, they were not paying for the treatments, so he stopped because he had no supporters.

## Snake Bite/Documentation

Elder Danjuma shared an incident that occurred during his shift while practicing. He narrated that a patient came to the hospital with a case of snakebite. "I admitted him, and I was trained never to give anti-snake venom directly but to give it slowly in dextrose saline and to observe the patient. The ward aid did not follow my instructions and administered the anti-snake poison directly. The patient died. I did not close on time because of this incident. I documented it, and it was the documentation that saved me. The hospital took over the case and explained everything to the patient's relatives.

This is a good lesson in nursing practice. Documentation is essential.

*If you don't have a good relationship with God, you will have relationship problems with people.*

◆ ◆ ◆

# CHAPTER 5

*Good Health*

Good health is living in harmony with God, others, oneself, and nature (the environment). "If there is a break in harmony in any of these relationships, then there is sickness." According to Stan Rowland, the restoration of disharmonious relationships is called "healing."

For you to live a joyful and healthy life, there are four crucial relationships you will need to build and maintain. These relationships are better made at a younger age before you advance and consider retirement. You will enjoy your retirement life because you developed a healthy relationship earlier.

## Harmony With God

To remain strong and healthy even in retirement, you must establish and maintain a good relationship with God, your creator. Know your God and live in obedience to his word and ordinances. Develop a consistent prayer life, speaking with God regularly and living a righteous life. It is essential at this moment to obey God's will in all you do, and you should keep praising him and giving him glory. In search of knowledge, look up to God for all your needs and submit totally to him. You should desire to please him and develop a hunger for the word of God.

Accept God's provision and trust him like babies trust their parents. Seek God's wisdom at all costs. God permits you to seek wisdom if you lack knowledge. He also says you should seek first his kingdom, and all other things will be added to you. Therefore, the first thing to look for is the word of God. Live as Jesus did. Jesus fed the people, healed many, provided for them, and helped them; he was disciplined, tested, visited, and empathized.

## Harmony With People

Sometimes it isn't easy to live with people. There are difficult neighbors all around. Make all efforts to live in peace with them. Keep obeying God's commandments by treating others well, regardless of their status. Being at peace with others is extremely helpful. Being relevant to them, showing love, and forgiving them are tools for healthy living. It is essential to obey the authorities that God has placed in leadership.

Make it a habit to give generously to meet the legitimate needs of other people. Consider getting involved in community service and initiating one where there is none, ensuring it is sustained. Get involved in advocacy as well. Speak for the voiceless and stand out for them. Ensure there is equity and justice in your vicinity. Advocate and speak for the voiceless.

> *When life on earth is ending, people don't surround themselves with objects. We want people around us—people we care about and with whom we have a relationship. In our final moments, we all realize that life is about relationships. Wisdom is learning that truth sooner than later. Don't wait until you die to figure out that nothing matters more.*
>
> Rick Warren

## Harmony With Self

No one will give you the happiness you desire. Many people cannot control their emotions, leading to the loss of relevant relationships that could be of value to them in later years. Make every effort to enjoy yourself and control your emotions. Make sure you are emotionally stable. Many people may see you and give an interpretation of who you are, based on their worldview. You should, however, try to see yourself in God's eye. How God sees you is what matters.

Understand who you are and what you can do best and keep doing it. Appreciate your weaknesses but try to effect necessary changes with time. You may reflect on your past life, which was not healthy and appreciative. Please forgive yourself and trust God to live a better life. Maintain good health emotionally, physically, socially, and spiritually. See that you can cope with adversity and disease. Ensure good hygiene, good habit, and a good attitude.

## Harmony With Nature (Environment)

Nature is the physical earth around us. The field's mountains, stones, and beasts are part of nature. God created the natural realm with laws that are in force for us to obey. The winds, earthquakes, etc., are part of the natural order. Throughout nature, viruses, bacteria, and parasites affect us. To be in good health, we must also live in harmony with the things around us. Most of our physical ill health is caused by living in disharmony with nature. Stripping our land of trees causes drought, erosion, and starvation. Pollution of our air and water causes many health problems. Respect God's land and animals. Don't destroy nature around us.

Human beings have a responsibility to protect the environment as stewards. Therefore, there should be a proper way of refuse disposal and landscaping. Conserve and develop God-given resources. Understand disease processes. Obey the laws of nature and take safety measures. Ensure good sanitation, take care of drainages, plant flowers and trees, and make a garden around you that is good for your health.

Good health is much more than just medical elements. It involves all facets of development which I will discuss here (Community Health Evangelism).

**Food:** Food is a significant component that every individual must have. You need more than just having food on your table. The body needs food that has all the nutrients to function and provide energy, nourishment, growth, etc. These also include excellent and clean water that will not introduce harmful organisms to your system, thereby causing various degrees of sickness to your body. People say that you are what you eat; therefore, know what you eat, how, and when to eat. Water, it is said, is life. Drink water regularly and take your time before you are testy. Water aids digestion and detoxifies your system. You become dehydrated when your body lacks water and exposes yourself to disease.

A Professor of Pharmacology, Mary O. Uguru cautions that you should avoid the following foods:
1. Refined and processed food.
2. Fatty food, fried food, and excessive animal proteins.
3. White rice, white bread, and other white flour products.
4. Artificial preservatives, flavors, colors, and stabilizers are added to processed foods.
5. Genetically engineered foods.

Oyedele Taye agrees with the above submission and adds that you should avoid late-night meals. She says that meals taken late at night usually do not get digested; therefore, take the last meal for the day 3 or 4 hours before bedtime.

**Medication:** Another necessity of life is medication. Unless otherwise stated, if one lives a good life, he will remain healthy. However, organ or system failure could occur as one ages. One apparent reason is that one loses millions of body cells daily as the body functions. The food we eat might not have enough nutrients our bodies need. Therefore often, time, he becomes ill and needs medication. There are numerous food supplements today to add up to what our daily food lacks.

Access to health care is essential, and if you patronize health insurance, it will help you. The National Health Insurance Authority (NHIA) is available for all individuals in Nigeria. Explore the possibility of being a partner and stakeholder.

**Education:** Education equips people with knowledge and skills. People get better jobs and earn more with a good education. Poverty is gone with a good education because higher wages will lead to lifelong learning. With more education, people learn to prevent disease; education also leads them to professional success. More education leads to healthier families and less malnutrition. Women with more education receive more care during their pregnancies and childbirth, so they have healthier babies. Education is a steppingstone to whatever one wants to do. It gives you a better social status and opens your eyes to opportunities. You don't have to depend on job opportunities; it helps create jobs.

**Friends**: Friends are people with similar interests. They are reliable and trustworthy, and they are always available. People say that "a friend indeed is a friend in need." A friend that cares shares their secret with you. They challenge and spur one another to get better in life. Shared interests form the core of friendship. If you have nothing to discuss to keep you together, you have nothing in common. Ensure that you make meaningful friends while in school. A songwriter says, "make new friends and keep the old. One is silver, and the other is gold." Learn to communicate well with friends and make good social connections.

Peace abounds in the absence of war, where people are free from war, and there is law and order. Freedom from public disturbance is evidence of peace. There is peace where there is no arguing or fighting between people but harmonious relationships, friendliness, and tranquillity. There is deceit in the hearts of those who plot evil but joy for those who promote peace. It is to a man's honor to avoid strife, but every fool is quick to quarrel. Try to be a person of peace. If you cannot be a part of the solution, do not harm or be a factor in the conflict.

**Emotional stability:** Anger is one sure way to show that one is not able to control their emotion. Therefore, learn how to manage your anger and humble yourself. Don't let anger cause you to sin; don't sleep with anger. Be gentle and patient with other people, bearing one another's doing. Do all things necessary to keep peace and unity together. Avoid evil and get rid of bitterness but build one another in love, kindness, and compassion. We are taught to confess to our brothers whenever we are angry with them, but not in an accusatory way.

The Bible also teaches that we should be quick to listen, slow to answer back, and slow to get angry. Taking the initiative to seek peace with another person when they have wronged you is essential. Forgive, forget, and don't hold a grudge against someone. As you age, avoid social isolation and withdrawal syndrome. Develop a stress coping mechanism and self-esteem. Exercise and rest are vital in your life.

**Rest:** Rest is an integral part of human beings. The importance of rest cannot be over-emphasized. Lack of rest can kill a relationship and cause stress to the individual. Rest reduces stress, boosts creativity, and improves productivity. Rest enhances decision-making, heals the body, and brings calmness, love, and care. The following are techniques to rest:

- Practice gratitude.
- Sleep is critical to survival.
- It is recommended for an adult to sleep 7-8 hours a day.
- Cultivate a healthy habit of exercise.
- Eat the right food at the right time.
- Prioritize activities.
- Plan rest in your diary.

- Rest after every project.
- Take time out with or without your family.
- There is time for everything.

The person that rests tend to do more work. Joy and happiness come only from within.

**Strong family**: There's no place like home. The home begins with the husband and his wife. The husband should respect the wife's body as physically weaker. The two should learn to share the workload in the home. Men, especially, are supposed to be doing the heaviest work. There should be sexual agreement and understanding of the needs of each other. They should be ready to listen to each other and agree on the pattern of kids' discipline. There should also be mutual respect and support while in pain and comfort in sorrow. Expressing feelings of love and appreciation and making decisions together are vital.

They should walk together in public while the husband protects his wife and helps her feel secure in dangerous places. They should not talk negatively about each other in public or with friends. One thing I do is inform my family about where I am going and when I am likely to return. Spiritually, both should desire to submit to God and spiritual elders, praying together and raising godly children. Take part in spiritual activities together, fellowships, home devotions, and studies. Serve the Lord together by helping the poor and needy, working in the community, and witnessing to friends and relations. Unity, networking, collaboration, and teamwork are essential for success. Don't neglect your family. See what Buehner Jan observes:

> *Aaron is Moses' older brother. Miriam is their sister.*
> *The three siblings follow similar careers and are connected through their family ties.*
> *Aaron is the spokesman for the brothers, even though Moses had a more vital calling and visionary powers.*
> *Miriam fulfils for the Israelite women a similar prophetic leadership role to that of her brothers.*

*She appears at the center stage from time to time.*

**Security:** Everybody needs security. Of course, security is a basic need. Security is a social system that ensures the safety of life and property. It is a state of being free from danger or threat. Where there is security, people follow rules and regulations. They are protected from harm. A financial asset is an excellent example of security. It will help if you prepare assets that have value and can be of use when finances are needed. Other types of security are food security, health security, physical security, economic security, environmental security, personal security, community security, and territorial security. Consult experts and invest in the best security you can for tomorrow.

**Faith:** The author of a fourteenth-century preacher's manual wrote that envy was "the most precious daughter of the devil because it follows his footsteps by hindering good and promoting evil." The author might have added that envy has a sister named malice, and the two usually work together. Envy causes inward pain when we see others succeed, and malice produces inward satisfaction when others fail. Envy and malice usually generate slander and unwarranted criticism. While these two sins hide behind the veil of religious zeal and self-righteousness, the poison they produce is even more deadly.

**Strengthen your devotion and prayer habits:** Continue in fellowship with brethren and communion. Try applying the biblical principles of humility, self-control, and compassion you learned from your Bible studies.

Very importantly, prayer is dependent on faith. It's like it doesn't exist without it, and it doesn't do anything if it's not accompanied. Faith makes prayer effectual, and in a certain important sense, must precede it," says E.M. Bounds.

*"Learning to forgive is vital to both our physical and mental well-being."*

◆ ◆ ◆

# CHAPTER 6

*Make Your Marriage Work*

Make your relationship more enjoyable to strengthen your bond daily. Determine in your heart that your marriage must work deliberately. You must introduce some practices to maintain a healthy and rewarding relationship. You may spice up your relationship and make it exciting for you and your partner to undertake it together; this can promote your health and prolong your life. Steve A. Adekanbi admonishes, "Marriage has to be a top priority." "Our relationship with our spouse should be the most important one on this earth."

Taking a trip with your spouse is a great way to spend quality time together while learning something new. To keep the love alive in your relationship, it's a good idea to go on a trip together, especially to places that interest your spouse. As such, the next time you contemplate strengthening your relationship, think about embarking on a journey with your lover.

Couples should learn and get involved in doing domestic and household duties together. They will be happier, supporting one another. It's a good idea to help your wife out around the house, such as cleaning up the dishes, putting away the furnishings, or taking care of the kids while she's doing other things. Assisting a lady will not only make her happy but also increase your status in her eyes.

For a relationship to thrive, both partners need to be involved in each other's daily lives in some capacity. To build a stronger relationship with your partner, you must engage in an active social life together. Relationships based on regular communication are more likely to last than those that are not.

To maintain good health, do not disregard the importance of intimacy in a relationship and playing indoor games. Couples should engage in various love activities to develop their relationship and improve their overall health. For example, couples can play hide-and-seek, truths or dares, pillow fights, water splashing, and even computer games. Playing these games with your partner will make your connection deeper and more enjoyable.

Visiting your spouse's hometown and immersing yourself in their values will instill a sense of purpose and mutual connection. Additionally, this might be an ideal date-night activity for couples on vacation.

Visiting an amusement park can be an excellent complement to the exciting activities that couples can do together. Experimenting with new outdoor activities, such as going to an amusement park with your lover, is one way to make your relationship more fun. Your relationship will benefit significantly if you and your partner engage in this type of bonding experience together.

Avoid any form of violence: physical, emotional, economic, sexual, and spiritual violence; it is not healthy in the home. Where any of the above exists, every family member is negatively affected, and the relationship becomes sour.

## Managing Money In The Home

Couples should learn to manage money as they grow older. At retirement, it will be less challenging for them. Dag Heward-Mills shares the following formula that will help manage money in the family:

1. Discuss money openly. Aim for transparency/openness in everything, especially in money matters.
2. Avoid selfishness
3. Note that you are only stewards of God's money.
    i. Spend it according to God's wishes and God's Word
    ii. You are accountable to Him.
4. Manage your finances properly by budgeting. These areas can guide you:
    i. God first (first and best fruits, offerings, tithes).
    ii. Savings and investment.
    iii. Address your NEEDS, not your wants.
    iv. Liabilities/obligations (debts, bills, remittances, blessing others). Extra (miscellaneous) to afford flexibility.
    v. Buying food in bulk saves money and reduces financial stress.

## Stress Management

Stress is pressure in our lives, and it comes from changes. The changes can be good or bad, positive, or negative. Positive stress may be the gift of a new car, the birth of a new baby, an unexpected promotion, a new job, etc. Negative stress can be anger, excess load, marginalization, the death of a loved one, etc. Other changes may be the suffering of a relative from a severe illness, dismissal from work, marriage, pregnancy, etc. Stress is a demand or pressure to which we must respond. Research shows that 75–90% of all diseases are stress related.

Stress can raise your blood pressure and cause diabetes, asthma, cancer, insomnia, etc. So the heart beats more quickly to pump more blood to the muscles and brain. Stress affects all areas of our lives, not just our bodies. Stress affects our thoughts, our emotions, our behavior, our spiritual lives, and our bodies.

Stress can cause broken homes, parental neglect, substance abuse, and many other ills if not managed well. The best way to manage stress is to try and take charge of your thoughts, emotions, schedules, and environment. Don't allow anyone to direct you.

## Tips For Managing Stress

- We can be open with God about our thoughts and our feelings.
- We can talk with a pastor or counselor.
- Exercise.
- Rest and relax.
- Eat well.
- Deep breath.
- Slow down.
- Take a break, meditate, and pray.
- Spend time in nature.
- Create time for hobbies.
- Talk about your problem.
- We can spend time with close friends.
- Eliminate stress triggers.

## Laughter For A Longer Life

*A cheerful heart does good, like medicine, but a broken spirit makes one sick. Proverbs 17:22.*

Rev. Prof. Musa A. Mambula believes that laughter has some healing properties, and he highlights the benefits below:
1. A Temporary Increase in Heart Rate: Improve blood circulation,

breathing, and muscle tone. Interestingly, this sounds like the benefits and results of physical exercise.

2. Lowered Blood Pressure and Pulse Rate As A Result Of The Exercise Ines the Nourishment Of Tissues: Healthy blood feeds the body better, which can also help prevent the formation of undesirable clotting.

3. Pain Reduction: This is often accompanied by less dependency on medication and shortened recuperation time from illness and surgical procedures. Laughter can also lessen the emotional pain.

4. Stress Reduction: Reducing the emission of the cortical hormones, which weaken the immune system, causes this.

5. Muscle Relaxation: This can ease the tension that breaks the spasm-pain cycle of rheumatism and neuralgia.

6. Increase Ventilation and Blood Oxygen Level: This can help people with emphysema and other respiratory illnesses. Laughter can assist in clearing mucus plugs.

7. Stimulation of the Immune System. One researcher found that watching a humorous video caused an increase in interferon-gamma both during and after the laughter experience, according to Mambula.

8. Sharpened Mental Functions: Jokes require attention. Word plays can keep the mind busy. Humor can stimulate the release of adrenaline and electrical activities.

9. Disease Isolation: Laughing together is a bonding experience. It is contagious, a socially transmitted disease of the best kind. It helps break down barriers among people and reduces hostility and conflict.

10. Decrease in Anxiety: It is difficult, if not impossible, to laugh and be afraid simultaneously.

11. Increased Ability to Cope: Being able to laugh with gusto can help people get through tough times, cope with the loss of good health, overcome grief, and get on with their lives.

12. Induction of Playfulness: Laughing can help people "regress" into a spirit of fun and adventure.

# Maturity

Are you immature? Learn to be mature. Are you foolish? Learn to have sense.

> *"Are you immature?" Learn to be mature. Are you foolish? "Learn to have sense."*
>
> Proverbs 8:5 (TEV)
>
> *"If any of you lacks wisdom, he should ask God, who gives generously to all without finding fault, and it will be given to him."*
>
> James 1:5 (NIV)

Maturity is when you can drop expectations from a relationship and give for giving sake. As you grow into adulthood, you must show various signs that you are mature.

Worshiping God is a good indicator of a spiritually mature person. Rev. Marcus Mayi Musa says, "worship is a sign of growth in the Lord because those who worship must be spiritually mature."

The following are signs of immaturity:
- They magnify Satan. Whatever you magnify manifests Psalm 68.
- They don't control their emotions.
- They think and behave like children.
- They find it difficult to accept others in their life and their understanding.
- They always think their knowledge is the best.

Mature people let go even when it hurts.
- Maturity is when you stop proving that you are right.
- Stop comparing yourself with others. Life is not a competition.
- You can't always get what you want.
- Be content and satisfied with your life while you aspire to higher heights.
- Maturity doesn't take revenge.

- Start thinking about others before yourself.
- You can't please everyone.
- See things from a different perspective than what you see immediately.
- Love more and judge less. Whoever does not love does not know God because God is love 1John 4:8.
- Pray for those who hate you.
- Appreciating your accomplishments, failures, destiny, reputation, and everything about your life depends on God's will and your choices, not pointing fingers at others.
- Maturity is the application of wisdom and knowledge and taking responsibility.
- Pursue kingdom matters: Knowing and serving God with all you have, no matter what people think or say.
- Immature Christians depend on carnal things as their testimonies.
- Immature Christians only remember God when the going is bad.
- Avoid instant gratification.

## The Cloud Of Worry

Many times, people live under what is called the "cloud of worry." Instead of addressing and attacking the real cause of the situation, they are overcome with worry. Koole describes worry as "the interest you pay on a debt you may never incur." According to Koole, the University of Michigan studied the things people worry about and discovered that more than 97 percent of all causes of worry are a waste of time. The result of their study goes thus:

60% of worries are unwarranted.

20% are past and unchangeable.

10% are too petty to waste your time on.

5% are unreal.

2½% are real, but you can't change them.

2½% are authentic and worthy of worry.

That means 97.5 percent of worry wastes time and other resources. They may appear factual, but they are just a cloud of worry. You can do without them. These statistics inform us that there is no need to worry.

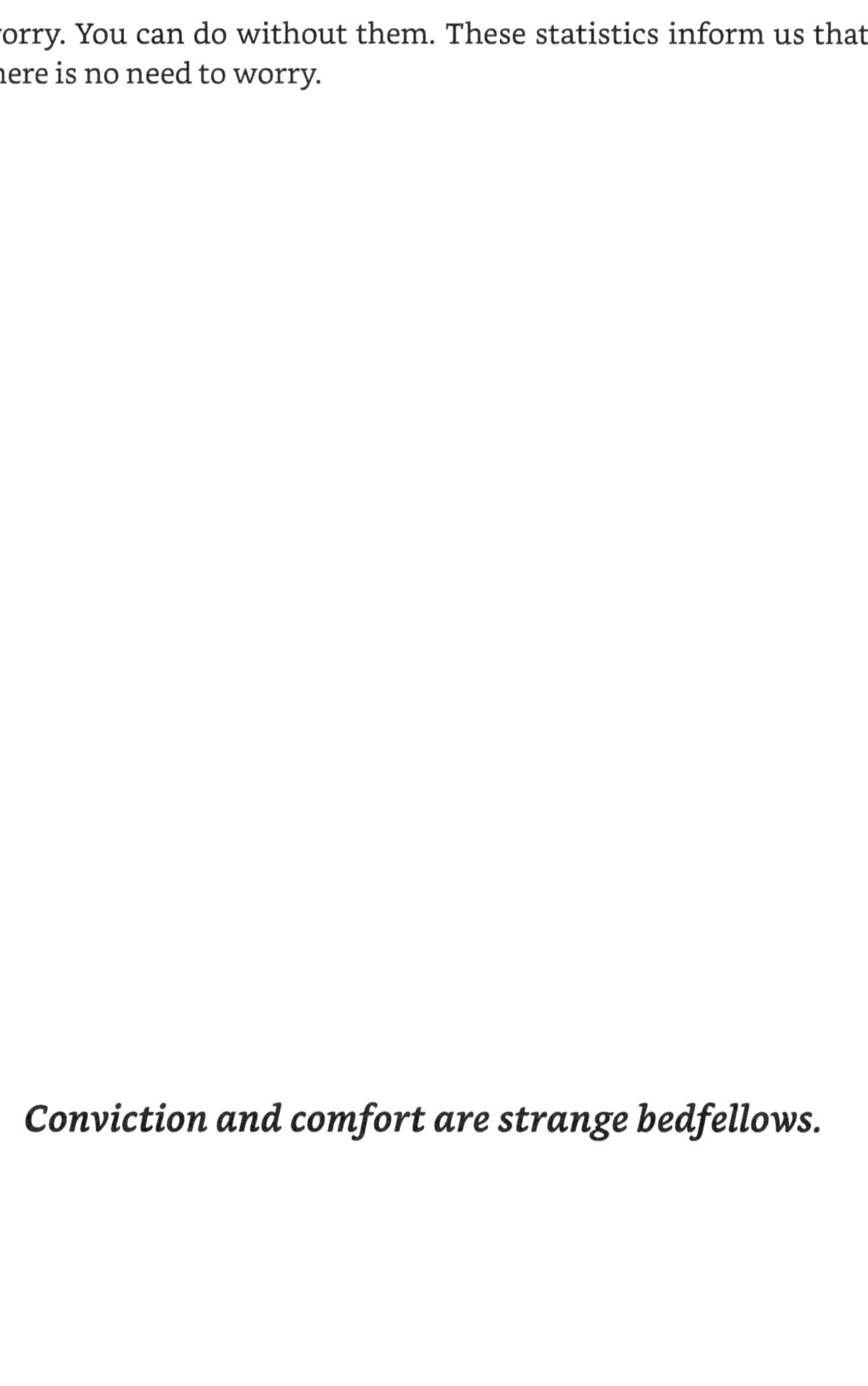

*Conviction and comfort are strange bedfellows.*

◆ ◆ ◆

# CHAPTER 7

*Overcoming Procrastination*

**M**any people have good plans but do not execute them because of procrastination. Sometimes it's laziness or a nonchalant attitude. The dangers of procrastination are enormous.

We are all familiar with the term "procrastination." When we procrastinate, we squander away our free time and put off important tasks we should be doing until it is too late. We regret and wish we could turn back the hands of time—the impossible.

**Definition**

Procrastination is the act of delaying or postponing an activity. It is unnecessarily and voluntarily delaying necessary action.

According to George S. Clason, you work hard to improve your skills and ensure a future income because wealth results from a reliable stream. You can only arrive at the peak of success once you crush the spirit of procrastination within you.

Those who procrastinate cannot meet deadlines. For instance, some students only submit their assignments once it becomes late.

You have a deadline looming. However, instead of doing your

work, you must catch up on inconsequential things like checking email and social media, watching videos, and surfing blogs and forums. You know you should be working, but you don't feel like doing anything.

## Why People Procrastinate

Why do we procrastinate, and, more importantly, what are the consequences, and what can we do about them?

There are several good reasons why people procrastinate. It could be, but is not limited to:

1. My mind is tired and needs some rest. I am trying to be patient and take care of myself. Let me sleep a bit and do it later.

2. I've had a lot on my table, which has been overwhelming. Not just work stuff (though there's lots of that), but family stuff. So instead of holding myself to impossible standards, I have to be compassionate and allow myself to create space, simplify, and find a path that works for me.

3. The fear of starting any task. For every new assignment, there is the fear of starting. One will always ask, "How can I even start?" When we think of work as something enormous, complex, stressful, overwhelming, or full of fear, procrastination sets in.

4. We avoid doing work to prevent our abilities from being criticized. And, if we succeed, we will feel much "smarter."

Everyone who says the above routinely procrastinates and has yet to complete an essential task for which they devised a strategy, implemented it, had time to review, and so on, before their deadline.

## Consequences Of Procrastination

The consequences of procrastination are enormous. Eleven of them are listed here:

1. Laziness
2. Feeling of anxiety
3. Stress
4. Fatigue
5. Disease
6. Disappointment
7. Producing below standard
8. Failure
9. Regret
10. Lost vision
11. Poverty

## Antidotes To Procrastination

What do we do to avoid procrastination? Leo Babauta shares four antidotes to procrastination.

## Antidote 1: Self-Care

The first thing to ask yourself if you're procrastinating is: "Am I tired?" "Do I need to take care of myself?" Find out if you are tired. You did so much work during the day and needed to rest.

The main ideas are to sleep, disconnect, get away from everything, and meditate. Reflect and contemplate. Once you're refreshed (which might mean a 20-minute nap and a short meditation), you can find mindful focus again.

## Antidote 2: Make A (Small) Commitment

Leo Babauta says, "What helped me during one point of my procrastination was to commit to a friend that I would do a bunch of work at a specific time. "And if I didn't do that work, I would have to suffer a consequence that we both agreed to."

When you commit to someone you respect, you'll elevate the act from something you want to shrink from to a vow you want to uphold. Then doing the work will be something you want to do.

Get a partner to whom you will be accountable, and both of you will agree.

## Antidote 3: Create The Space

A big part of the problem with constant procrastination is that we are in an environment conducive to distraction and doing small, inconsequential tasks (like checking messages, answering emails, seeing how many likes you got on Facebook, etc.)

You might brace yourself to do the work but then decide to check one thing quickly, which leads to checking another. And before you know it, a whole day has gone by. It's hard to focus when you're in an environment like this.

Turn off Wi-Fi, set up an Internet blocker, unplug your router, or get somewhere where there is no Internet. With an environment like this, you will be able to focus much better.

## Antidote 4: Find The Joy In It

Develop love and joy for what you decide to do. Your attention will always be there, and you will make every effort to accomplish it. So, a switch in mindset would be hugely beneficial. If you love doing it, you won't procrastinate!

Consider your job to be a treasured activity that you are privileged to do because only a few people get to do it. Your brain will start to program itself to dive into this joyful activity, and you will be awake to the world.

## Practical Ways To Stop Procrastinating

Celestine Chua is the founder of Personal Excellence. She gives her best advice on how to stop procrastination, boost productivity, and achieve excellence.

Don't let procrastination take over your life. Here are steps on how to stop procrastinating:

1. Break Your Work into Little Steps
2. Change Your Environment
3. Create a Detailed Timeline with Specific Deadlines
4. Eliminate Your Procrastination Pit-Stops
5. Reduce the Number of Decisions You Need to Make Throughout the Day
6. Finish Your Day Before It Starts
7. Re-Clarify Your Goals
8. Stop Over-Complicating Things
9. Reward Yourself
10. Give Yourself a Break
11. Hang out with People Who Inspire You to Act
12. Get Motivation, Buddy
13. Tell Others About Your Goals
14. Seek out Someone Who Has Already Achieved the Outcome

According to Celestine Chua, chronic procrastinators spend years looping in this cycle, delaying, putting things off, slacking off, hiding from work, and facing tasks only when inevitable, then repeating this loop all over again. It's a bad habit that eats us away and prevents us from achieving more remarkable results in life.

I have never heard anyone procrastinate their way to success before,  and I wonder if it will change soon. Whatever you are procrastinating, if you want to get it done, you need to get a grip on yourself and do it.

*Love is not a good part of your life;
it's the most critical part.*

# CHAPTER 8

## *Home and Responsibilities in the Family*

A home is a place where the family dwells. Gordon McDonald asserts, "There's no place like home if those in charge care passionately for the moral and spiritual messages allowed in the door." The family is an independent institution where shared responsibilities abound. For the family to stand, each person must take their responsibilities seriously.

A happy family is one where love binds people together. Crowford W. Loritts insists that you should never walk away from responsibilities. Family members should take their responsibility seriously and be committed to them.

The children have two significant roles to play in the family.

1. At an early age, they need to obey their parents.
2. At a later age, they must take good care of their aging parents.

Couples, on the other hand (in some families), are in pain instead of experiencing the desired pleasure. This could result from a lack of knowledge on either or both sides.

Many parents go to early graves out of disappointments and regrets they experience because of the misconception about the role their children should play in their later years.

The world is dynamic and changing, but some people don't know that. Beliefs are changing to suit the new era of technology. The microwave mindset and the jet-age syndrome are fast turning our beliefs against us.

For instance, today, it is an error for parents in the village to choose a wife for their son in the city. It was, however, the practice many decades ago in Africa. Furthermore, the concept of raising a male child, mainly the firstborn, with the intention of him working and training his siblings is gradually fading away. Training a child and expecting them to care for you in old age proves to be a mistake.

In the 21$^{st}$ century, parents must develop a new formula for training their children and then plan for their later years to avoid becoming a burden or eating the food of sorrow.

At every phase of life, demand differs. Besides good health and a sound mind, positive cash flow cuts across every stage of life. Lack of positive cash flow compounds problems at every phase, particularly at a later age. The more one advances in age, the more one needs.

Considering health, for example, some people become weak at forty to fifty, and the need to maintain the body arises. More so if any body organ is failing, you must employ medical aid, which costs money. Your ability to afford medical bills guarantees you a seasoned doctor. Otherwise, you patronize a chemist with no doctor's prescription and wonder what you're buying.

Neatness in terms of clothing is another issue. You will need laundry services. The cost of materials and serving is rising daily.

Your eating habit must change. To be on the safe side, you need the advice of a dietician.

Then your daily essentials. The cost of maintaining the home and replacing your household items is also high; you will need all these things. The question is, how often will you rely on your children for all of these?

Unless you are among the early starters whose children have completed their education by the time the parents are in their fifties, it's when the children are not too busy with the challenges of the present age.

So, we can see that the older you become, the more cash you need to keep your body and soul together. In a country like Nigeria, some grandchildren are still being taken care of by grandparents who are already retired. This can be a pressure point in retirement. It would save everyone the hassles of education expenses if they planned all of this.

Retirement can be much more fun if there is a lot of money to spend. Though you don't need to amass huge funds to retire comfortably, careful planning can leave you with enough money to enjoy your retirement in peace.

How about your children's university education, graduation, establishing their trade, wedding ceremonies, etc.? All these are financially demanding if you are a parent worth your salt. These are some of the responsibilities. Does it mean that today's children are not compassionate or merciful, or do they not know their duties towards their parents? No.

In our society today, by the time your child finishes his education, they desire a reliable source of income to start a family. At this point, your phase of life and demands are different. As a responsible parent, you would like to see your child meet the needs of their generation; at the same time, you would like to meet up with your peer group.

In another development, the youths' problems and challenges today differ from what they were about thirty years ago. Today, the youth must be more creative and have a sound education. They must create jobs and legitimate means of income to sustain themselves with what they have learned. The days of abstract knowledge are gone; creativity must be added to the abstract for your education to have a whole meaning.

Suddenly, we discover that classroom knowledge offers you a certificate rather than a befitting job. Some parents today spend extra money on their children so that they can compete favorably in the competitive labor market. Opportunities are available for those with additional intelligence and creative grace, which are not available in the general classroom. So, youths face difficult times in meeting life's demands.

With the above challenges, the only guarantee for children to care for their aging parents is if the parents maintain a source of income.

Many parents succeed with this agenda, while many die with regret and disappointment because they failed to realize that times have changed.

## Make Sure You Are Not Financially Dependent On Your Children.

Getty Image shares certain things to avoid so that you will not be financially reliant on your children at retirement.

Children in the 21$^{st}$ century live far away to pursue careers that their parents don't fully comprehend. Parents, you must set aside funds to live an independent retirement to avoid disappointment. There are exceptions. However, people's ideas are changing about how much they can depend on their grown children. Before the 21$^{st}$ century, children solely cared for the elderly.

In Africa, particularly, we remain culturally tied to the ideas of sacrifice, servitude, and homage to elders, and we celebrate dependence as a mark of communal living. Grown-up children continue to live with their parents; grandparents actively bring up their grandchildren, and parents expect their children to look after them when the circumstance warrants it.

However, the reality is that these expectations are costly. They require a lot of resources, time, and effort, which may be offered with simmering resentment, as experienced by some of us.

To avoid this, you must prioritize your old age comfort and make sure you have provision for it. If you have a house of your own, continue to keep and live in it during your time.

Getty Image says you should "recognize that your life stage and your children's are very different." "As a retired person, you have all the time; you have limited responsibilities towards others; and you may be secure with your funds for the future." "Your children have their careers to chase, children to raise, and homes to build. Depending on them for time, attention, and resources can be draining for them and create resentment." "Rely on your circle of like-minded friends and keep doing what you are used to instead." "Find a purpose beyond hanging out with your grown-up children and their families."

In addition, your children would love and care for you and would be willing to support you if you could take care of your regular routines without demanding their time. Speak to them about your fears and apprehensions and get them to commit to helping with what might be genuinely challenging for you to deal with alone. They will be happier to visit often, and it will be easier for them to render help.

Avoid feeling entitled to the wealth of your children. We could demand that they remain grateful for what we did for them when we brought them up, but they are busy bringing up their children. My father used to say that whatever his children did to him was just an attempt to pay back what he had spent on them. One day, one of my siblings jokingly asked him to calculate all he had spent on him so he could pay upfront. Seek the children out as an exception rather than as a norm. They have their priorities for their income, and you must not grudge that; it's a reality.

## What To Do

    **1.** Work at having multiple streams of income that

will stand the test of time. Get involved with financial experts for counsel on investment. However, be careful to avoid falling into the wrong hands. Many people have become victims of fraud and were disappointed at further investments.

2. Plan your life so that you are responsible for yourself until you breathe your last breath. Commitment goes with action. Be prepared to be active at whichever age. By so doing, you will enjoy good health and longevity.

3. Show love and affection to your children and your spouse. Teach your children how to give gifts. You expect your children to grow to love and appreciate you. Therefore, demonstrate love to them so they will not forget. Love your spouse and let them know that their parents love each other. Whatever I did to my parents while they lived, I did it in the presence of my children to see. The idea is that when they grow up, they will also remember me. When I am old and withdrawn from active service, they will know they have a responsibility.

4. Budgeting on another man's purse is setting up for disgrace. Do not depend on anybody, no matter how close you are to the person. Don't even depend on your children. If they come visiting, good; if they don't, trust God to sustain your investment. The children will also be facing the challenges of their own time.

5. Seek God and pray for your children. Develop a habit of praying for your children as Job would do:

When a period of feasting had run its course, Job would send and have them purified.
Early in the morning, he would sacrifice a burnt offering for each of them, thinking,

**Perhaps my children have sinned and cursed God in their hearts. This was Job's regular custom.**

Job 1:5 (NIV).

According to Gordon MacDonald, there's no place like home if each person knows they belong and are bonded to the family unconditionally. In a home, family members rely on one another with full hope. Sometimes hope comes true; other times, there are disappointments. With increased uncertainties, each person should develop themselves and trust God to end strong.

## Case Study Of Emmanuel Onwe Akpo

Emmanuel Onwe Akpo is *married to Choice Emmanuel Akpo, with children.* He **was trained as a teacher** but went into full-time mission work with students under The Fellowship of Christian Students (FCS), Nigeria. He served between 1994 and 2013 and **retired in 2013** from FCS National Headquarters after serving eight years as National Director. In all, he worked in FCS for 19 years.

Emmanuel Onwe Akpo retired because he was convinced to do so, having served in various capacities, from being a field staff member (Training Secretary) to the Chief Executive of the organization. I depended on God to guide me on the proper time to retire, and He did. So, I responded to divine guidance.

*"I believe in retiring strong and vibrant. I retired at 51 years old."*

This is important so as not to be a burden or a liability in the workplace, as is the common experience in government and nongovernmental organizations today. Retiring when one is still strong makes room for venturing into new areas as God guides. "Even if one makes mistakes, there will be the strength to make changes or a complete U-turn," according to Emmanuel Akpo.

## Challenges Associated With Retirement

Often, retirement is not pleasant for several reasons, as

highlighted by Emmanuel Akpo:

i. Fear of unknown
ii. No previous savings to fall back on
iii. No personal (house) accommodation, and thus how to cope with paying rent.
iv. Children's education if they are still in school.
v. Family upkeep
vi. How to respond to social demands. Strength to cope with new challenges in the "new world."
vii. Inability to think creatively to see and explore other opportunities for services beyond the familiar terrain.
viii. Concern for prestige and what people will think about you and your new source of income.
ix. Poor or lack of retirement benefits and a lot more, depending on the individuals and the type of organization.
x. Poor or lack of training to equip staff for retirement.

No one is immune to these concerns. It's, therefore, imperative to trust God when confronted with the need to retire. This was Emmanuel's situation when he retired, trusting God for the next step since he didn't have any solid retirement plans.

"For the past nine years of retirement, I have every reason to thank God for following and trusting His leadership. I have never regretted any that I had to retire."

## What Did I Do Then And Now?

As soon as he disengaged, he got involved in multilevel marketing (MLM). This gave him great satisfaction as he saw it as another dimension of ministry. He reached hundreds of people with fantastic products that were effective in their lives and families. "Even though it was a humbling service, I was never ashamed despite mockery and criticism from so-called concerned individuals who were never supportive." That humble service gave me an economic quantum lift that enabled me to own a house in Jos and my village. TO GOD BE THE GLORY FOR THE GREAT THINGS HE HAS DONE FOR MY FAMILY," asserted Emmanuel Akpo.

By 2015, Emmanuel Akpo volunteered and served with Doulos Education Enterprises, the Legal representative of Accelerated Christian Education (ACE), USA, in Nigeria. He was saddled with the responsibility of coordinating ACE training in Nigeria. This gave him another higher level of satisfaction, gradually allowing him to disengage from MLM. It afforded him the opportunity of diverse training using another educational curriculum which opened his eyes to other doors of opportunity. By 2016, he began home schooling his children, which had many benefits that I cannot describe here.

Furthermore, the Home School became the nucleus of a formal school that took off in 2017 to date. "Now, my wife and I are running a school (Royal Choice Christian School, RCCS, Jos) using the ACE curriculum. To the glory of God, our first son has graduated from the same school. What a great privilege it is to disciple children for the Kingdom. "Here is our ideal destination, except God leads otherwise."

## Project Supporters

Besides God, his wife and children are the most significant supporters Emmanuel Akpo has ever had. God also raised innumerable individuals who supported him at different times in different places to bring him to where he is today.

## Counsel From Emmanuel Akpo

1. Every employee should plan for retirement right from the first year of employment.
2. Keep your usefulness and productivity high.
3. Trust God to make you realize when your time is up.

Don't just hang on for economic benefits or fear of the unknown. The just shall live by faith.

4. There may be far better opportunities elsewhere if you care to listen to God.

5. Determine to be an employer of labor and not die an employee. Don't be content with earning salaries no matter how much. Salaried work is a social bondage.

6. Sharpen your skills and seek to acquire new ones to respond to the changes in our ever-changing world. Only those who respond to changes readily and efficiently can become agents of change.

Another thing I notice about Emmanuel Akpo is that he involves his family members in any project he embarks on, enhancing their maximum cooperation, active support, and understanding. Such is the case with Aaron, Moses, and Mariam in the Bible.

## Case Study Of Rev. Ishaya Manami

Rev. Ishaya Manomi retired from active service with the Church Of Christ In Nations (COCIN) in 2016 upon reaching 65. He served the church for 32 years and retired in Mwari in Bogoro Local Government Area of Bauchi State, Nigeria. He has seven children with his wife, Mama Rhodah Manomi. They have grandchildren and are all doing well.

Farming is their mainstay now, though Rev. Ishaya Manomi maintains that sometimes he only farms to his satisfaction if there is money for labor. He says, at retirement, the strength is no longer there to farm rigorously. He also says that his children greatly help him at this retirement age. They are now his major supporters in life.

## Counsel

Rev. Ishaya Manomi counsels that:

1. Young people should marry at the appropriate age, so they do not have to train children when they retire. When you are older and have less strength, the children will also support you.
2. They should also try to build their residence before retiring because, at retirement, there is a meager income.

## Advantages Of Retirement

The challenge of retirement is that the rewards and support from the church cease. However, there are no more trips; therefore, one has enough time to rest and carry out some private commitments at will, according to Rev. Ishaya Manomi.

## Power Of Prayer

We cannot overemphasize the power of prayer. Gyang Pam insists that we should pray and confess our sins. He says, "Nothing keeps us from our creator like our sins." The prayer of confession is one of the most vital prayers we have. It involves one acknowledging his sin, shortcoming, and weakness before Go." Ezekiel Dachomo agrees with Gyang Pam and adds, "A prayer of confession is a way of acknowledging and repenting from our sin."

> *If we confess our sins, he is faithful and just to forgive us and cleanse us from all unrighteousness.*
>
> (1 John 1:9).

Sarah K. Mavirah shared her widowhood experience and concluded that prayer sustained her. She says prayer is her life's wire, and she cannot live without it.

## Conclusion

This book was born out of passion and desire to help people of all works of life to plan and live a meaningful life after retirement.

I see many people retire poor and suffer from different untold hardship. Many of them develop organ failure or a terminal illness; some eventually die too soon after retirement. The reasons for all these are examined in this book. There are notable solutions that will be of help to many who are able to access this book. Selected retirees who are doing well after retirement were interviewed to share their success stories. This will encourage others to also plan well and prepare for retirement to reduce the ugly unexpected. This book is just an introductory part of series about retirement that will follow suit. Watch out!

# WORKS CITED


Abraham Tativ. Interview. Gboko 4th January 2023

Adekanbi, A. Steve (2019). Strategic Mentoring for Outstanding Success. Christheirs Nigeria ventures.

Ajiboye, Richard Dare (2020). Fixing Your Retirement Before Retiring. Richard Dare Ajiboye Adebowale House.

Akpo, Emmanuel Onwe. Questionnaire. Zarmaganda, Jos. 26th December 2022.

Alamba, Timothy. The Light Bearer. Church Of Christ in Nations (June 2021).

Bounds, E.M. (2010). Necessity of Prayer. Revival Publishing.

Buba, Hosea G. Questionnaire. Maiduguri, 27th December 2022.

Burial Program: Ngo Victoria Yop Yaro Bot Davou. 28th December 2022.

Clason, George S. (2007). The richest Man in Babylon. Glorious Life Publications.

Dachomo, B. Ezekiel (2022). The Power of Prayer in The Daily Life of A Christian. Theo Koncept Publishers.

Dali, Rebecca Samuel (2007). Wealth Creation and Savings: Some Biblical Principles and Ethics. Baraka Press and Publishers Limited.

Dastu, R. Ring-le. Interview. Munchogopiom, Jos 4th January 2023

Dawang, Joel. Interview. Zarmaganda, Jos 11th September 2022.

Dawang, Sarah. Interview. Zarmaganda, Jos. 11th September 2022.

Dikko, Hannatu. Interview. Zarmaganda, Jos 17th October 2022.

Gomiyar, Joel. The Light Bearer. Church Of Christ in Nations (May 2021).

Heward-Mills Dag (2012). Model Marriage: A Marriage Counseling Handbook. Hosanna Christian Bookshop & Publishing.

http://opr.news/s29fd183e221222en_ng?link=1&client=news

https://www.actsretirement.org/retirement-resources/resources-advice/what-to-do-in-retirement/3-types-of-retirement/

Ijaopo, O. Isaac (2006). Family Financial Empowerment. Help-Line Publications.

Ishaya Manomi. Interview. Mwari, Bogoro, 4th January 2023

Izekor, Victor. The Light Bearer. Church Of Christ in Nations (June 2022).

Izekor, Victor. The Light Bearer. Church Of Christ in Nations (March 2022).

Jan, Buehner (2003). Health and Wholeness: Healing Stories From The Bible, Thomson Press, India.

Kiyosaki and Lechter (2002). Rich Dad's Guide To Investing What The Rich Invest in That The Poor and Middle Class Do Not. Warner Books in Association with CASHFLOW Technologies, Inc.

Koole, Richard. Outsmarting Stress: Biblical Principles for handling Life's Pressure. Edysyl Publications.

Loritts, Crowford W. (1997). Never Walk Away: Lessons on Integrity From a Father Who Lived It. Moody Press, Chicago

Maisaini, Alexander Usman (2009). Poverty Is a Choice: Biblical Principles of Overcoming Poverty in Africa. Wisdom Books Publications.

Malkmus, George H. (2005). Why Christians Get Sick. Destiny Image Publishers.

Mambula, Musa A (2006). Leadership and Storms of Stress: How to

Overcome It. Baraka Press & Publishers Ltd, Kaduna.

Mavirah, K. Sarah (2010). Victory In Adversity. Larigraphics Printers.

McDonald, Gordon (1991). There's no Place Like Home. Tyndale House Publishers, Inc, Wheaton, Illinois.

Musa, Marcus Mayi (2010). Christian Worship. Marcus M. Musa.

Mufuyai, Hajiya Kadiza, Interview. Mangu, Plateau State 20th January 2023.

Nwan, Timothy (2009) The Integrity of a Name. Timceli Ventures Nigeria.

Oyedele, Taye (2008). Staying Healthy Through Proper Dieting. Favour Dietary Consult.

Pam, David Gyang (2008). Pray Again. Niri Press

Rowland, Stan (2001). Multiplying Light & Truth Through Community Health Evangelism. Printed & Bound in India.

Uguru, Mary O. (2007). Diet, Herbs & Holistic Health. Larigraphics, Jos.

Warren, Rick (2002). The Purpose Driven Life. Oasis International LTD.

www.economictimes.com Getty Image, 6thealed.com

www.moringarevealed.com

# ABOUT THE AUTHOR

**Rev. Simeon Terhemen Kaase**

had a semi-retirement voluntarily from the Nigeria Police Force after 17 years of service. He now works with the Fellowship of Christian Nurses, Nigeria and he is the Director of Missions. He coordinates to concept of Faith Community Nursing in Nigeria.

He is a Theologian and holds a Bachelor of Divinity (BD) from the Theological College of Northern Nigeria (TCNN), Bukuru and BA in Christian Religion, University of Jos, Plateau State. He holds Advance Diploma in Public Admin (ADPA) and he is also a Registered Nurse.

Rev. Simeon Terhemen Kaase is a Master trainer, facilitator and Practitioner of Community Health Evangelism (CHE), a community development and transformation strategy. He is a trainer of Saline Witness Process. He is into mentoring young people to prepare them in making informed decision in life.

He bagged Distinction and was awarded the Most Industrious Male BY THE MANAGEMENT OF WRITE-FOR-ME. He lives in Jos with his wife Mrs. Veronica Kaase and children.

# ABOUT THE BOOK

This book was born out of passion and desire to help people of all works of life to plan and live a meaningful life after retirement. Some people retire and suffer from organ failure or a terminal illness; some eventually die too soon after retirement. The reasons for all these are examined in this book. Selected retirees who are doing well after retirement were interviewed to share their success stories. This will encourage others to also plan well and prepare for retirement to reduce the ugly unexpected. This book is just an introductory part of series about retirement that will follow suit. Watch out!

www.ingramcontent.com/pod-product-compliance
Lightning Source LLC
Chambersburg PA
CBHW061324250726
48657CB00016B/532